Wellness Made Simple

WELLNESS MADE SIMPLE

PATSY NEAL

Kroshka Books
Commack, New York

Editorial Production: Susan Boriotti
Office Manager: Annette Hellinger
Graphics: Frank Grucci and John T'Lustachowski
Information Editor: Tatiana Shohov
Book Production: Donna Dennis, Patrick Davin, Christine Mathosian, Tammy Sauter and Diane Sharp
Circulation: Maryanne Schmidt
Marketing/Sales: Cathy DeGregory

Library of Congress Cataloging-in-Publication Data available upon request.

ISBN 1-56072-477-3

Copyright © 1999 by Patsy Neal
  Kroshka Books, a division of
  Nova Science Publishers, Inc.
  6080 Jericho Turnpike, Suite 207
  Commack, New York 11725
  Tele. 516-499-3103   Fax 516-499-3146
  e-mail: Novascience@earthlink.net
  e-mail: Novascil@aol.com
  Web Site: http://www.nexusworld.com/nova

All rights reserved. No part of this book may be reproduced, stored in a retrieval system or transmitted in any form or by any means: electronic, electrostatic, magnetic, tape, mechanical photocopying, recording or otherwise without permission from the publishers.

The authors and publisher haven taken care in preparation of this book, but make no expressed or implied warranty of any kind and assume no responsibility for any errors or omissions. No liability is assumed for incidental or consequential damages in connection with or arising out of information contained in this book.

This publication is designed to provide accurate and authoritative information with regard to the subject matter covered herein. It is sold with the clear understanding that the publisher is not engaged in rendering legal or any other professional services. If legal or any other expert assistance is required, the services of a competent person should be sought. FROM A DECLARATION OF PARTICIPANTS JOINTLY ADOPTED BY A COMMITTEE OF THE AMERICAN BAR ASSOCIATION AND A COMMITTEE OF PUBLISHERS.

Printed in the United States of America

Contents

Foreword	vii
Preface	ix
Acknowledgments	xiii

PART I   A LOOK AT WELLNESS

Introduction to Chapter 1		3
Chapter 1	Wellness...What Is It?	5
Introduction to Chapter 2		13
Chapter 2	The Awesome Mind and Body	15

PART II   WHAT'S KILLING US?

Introduction to Chapter 3		29
Chapter 3	So Why Are Our Awesome Bodies Dying Young?	31

PART III   HOW DO I IMPROVE MY HEALTH?

Chapter 4	The Big Ten	45
Chapter 5	Other Big Principles	67

PART IV A CLOSER LOOK AT A HEALTHY LIFE

Introduction to Chapters 6-10   101

Chapter 6   Positive Relationships   103

Chapter 7   Stress Management   107

Chapter 8   Sexual Responsibility   113

Chapter 9   Living With Our Environment   119

Chapter 10   Staying Morally and Spiritually Well   127

PART V WHERE DO I GO FROM HERE?

Introduction to Chapters 11-13   135

Chapter 11   Establishing A Plan of Action   137

Chapter 12   Growing Older, Getting Healthier   147

Chapter 13   Keeping Wellness Simple   163

FOREWORD

Even though our knowledge of wellness has increased, the health habits of many Americans have become worse over the last decade. While one-fourth of our nation was overweight in the early 60's, this number has increased to over one-third in the 90's. At the same time, according to a recent Surgeon General's report, only 22% of Americans get the minimum 30 minutes regular exercise that is suggested for good health.

Despite excellent programs such as "Healthy People 2000" and the millions of dollars spent on research and education, and despite widespread knowledge that good health habits can decrease the risk of heart disease, diabetes, high blood pressure, certain forms of cancer, obesity, and other life-threatening illnesses, a majority of Americans continue to choose lifestyle habits that take away from their quality of life.

We must take our health more seriously. Even though most of us know that there are specific things we can do to reduce our risks of poor health and premature death, few of us are truly committed to this type of life-long, healthy lifestyles.

It is time for us to take a long, hard look at what poor health is doing to us, not only as individuals, but to our economy and our American way of life.

This book, WELLNESS MADE SIMPLE, can serve as a road-map for you. It not only defines the ten leading causes of deaths in the United States, and tells you how you can decrease your risk factors, but it will give you invaluable information on where you can obtain help in breaking bad health habits...and best of all, it will motivate you to look at your body and mind in a new light.

If all of us could make just a few simple changes in our lifestyles, it would not only save our nation billions of dollars, but it would make us all happier, healthier, and more productive individuals.

Please take time to read WELLNESS MADE SIMPLE, and incorporate the key principles of health into your lifestyle.

>Robert F. Burgin
>President & CEO
>Mission St. Joseph's Health System

PREFACE

This book is about wellness...but it is about much more than that. It is about life and living...about improving the quality of your existence by feeling better, stronger, fitter, and more confident.

It is not like most books you will pick up on Wellness. This book has been written to help busy people get to the principles of good health as quickly as possible, so they can go about the business of living their lives.

This book is unique in that it focuses on the ten leading causes of death in the United States, and how the individual can cut his/her risk of dying from one of these leading causes of death.

With the rising costs of health care, few of us can afford the luxury of neglecting our health. Recently, it was estimated that 1.3 million Americans would die prematurely in a year's time. In 1988 alone, the nation faced a $600 billion expenditure for medical care, more than $1,900 per person. By 1993, it had jumped to $3,299 for every man, woman, and child, or a total of $884 billion dollars (about 13.9 percent of the gross domestic product). In the year 2000, it has been predicted that the per person annual health care costs could escalate to $5,500.

As we get older, health problems may intensify. One study found that almost half of all nursing home patients are given the wrong prescription drugs, oftentimes resulting in adverse reactions (one-third of adults over 65 take eight or more prescribed drugs daily).

Each of us must be more conscious of our everyday habits and how much we control our lifespan and the quality of our lives.

To be healthier, it is not necessary that we know all the research that has been done on the subject of Wellness, or know about all the complex interactions of our body. It is necessary that we know what works and what does not work, and that we recognize there are certain timeless, steadfast principles of good health that remain constant. These principles work just as well when stated simply as when written in complicated and scientific language.

So, this book is not written to impress you. It is written to help you. To do so, it has purposely been written in an easily understood form, without confusing charts and graphs.

This does not mean this book is not comprehensive. It gives you everything you need to know to help you stay well, but all the "fat" has been taken away from the overwhelming, immense volume of material on the market in order to give you the vital "meat." Consequently, the confusion has been stripped away from dealing with too much information.

Key points, brief statements, and general guidelines will give you an overall view of each specific component of wellness. If you should need more information, you can refer to the list of selected readings.

Something you should find extremely helpful are the web sites and phone numbers of organizations that can help you with lifestyle changes. Most of the phone numbers are toll-free.

I have attempted to add a very special human dimension to these pages, for I know from my personal experience as a three-time All-American athlete and as an instructor of Health, Physical Education, and Recreation for twenty-one years that there is a lot more to life than facts and tangible knowledge.

Even though I want you to know the mechanics and techniques of stress management, weight control, and all the other components of wellness...I especially want you to know the joy of fitness and the incredible feelings of having your body and mind respond well to the constant demands of everyday living.

I want you to fall in love with Wellness...with the way good health makes you feel. I want you to see that Wellness is not just a nice thing to have happen to you, but that you have the power to obtain it through your own personal decisions and choices, and that it is essential to your total well-being. And I especially want you to know how magnificent the human body really is.

We are amazing beings, with the capacity to live wonderful, creative, productive and healthy lives. However, the spirit can not soar if the physical body drags it down, nor can the body do incredible feats if the mind is not working effectively, or the spirit is not willing. We limit ourselves greatly when any part of our totality does not operate properly.

Our health is affected by almost everything, so the concept of Wellness is encompassing. Working on only one part of our health, such as losing weight or becoming fit, will not get the job done. To give us full benefits, the search for Wellness must pervade every part of our being and become one of the top priorities of our lives. Living well should be our goal, and well living should be our quest in life.

One beautiful thing about Wellness, as you will see in the chapter on "Growing Older, Getting Healthier," is that it is never too late to reap some of the benefits of a positive lifestyle.

In our fast-paced society, there are so many things we can not control in our lives. It is comforting to know that usually we can affect the way we feel by our daily decisions and choices. It is also comforting to know that Wellness is really fairly simple when we know how to pursue it.

We are each so different, yet each of us is so similar in our need to find happiness and satisfaction in our lives. Constantly, we are all searching for a better way of life. This book, WELLNESS MADE SIMPLE, was written to help you in your search to become a vibrant, happy, healthy human being.

I wish you well in your pursuit of good health and quality living.

ACKNOWLEDGMENTS

I would like to thank Tom Forkner, Manager, Franklin (N.C.) Health and Fitness Center, and Alisa Krizan, Cardiac Dietician, Mayo Clinic, for their review and helpful comments on my manuscript.

I would also like to thank Debbie Sprouse for her ideas and help, and my family and friends for their encouragement and support during the writing of this book.

PART 1

A LOOK AT WELLNESS

Look to your health; and if you have it, praise God...

- Izaak Walton

Introduction to Chapter 1

A wise man should consider that health is the greatest of human blessings...
- Hippocrates

When you really think about it, there is nothing more important than good health. Our happiness, our productivity, our emotional and mental well-being, our creativity, our ability to cope with life, and oftentimes our finances, are all connected to how we feel.

We all wish to be well. When something goes wrong with our health, it makes life more difficult. It is when we have a positive relationship with our bodies, our neighbors, and our surroundings that life is a pleasure and all seems well with the world. We seek wellness because it gives our life balance.

Almost everything we do and everything we come into contact with, affects our health in some way. Wellness consists of so many dimensions that oftentimes, we overlook parts of our lives that keep us healthy and happy. Some things we need to constantly be aware of that affect our health are sound relationships, intellectual and spiritual growth, emotional fulfillment, environmental interaction, and a strong, fit body that works smoothly with a healthy mind, spirit, and social consciousness.

Often we may have to make sacrifices because a state of wellness is in opposition to other things that give us pleasure (if we believe that good nutrition is vital to our well-being, we may have to give up some of the foods we enjoy).

Good health and wellness is truly a blessing, and is obtainable when we keep all the dimensions of our life balanced.

CHAPTER 1

WELLNESS...WHAT IS IT?

WHAT DO I NEED TO KNOW?

- There is no one single definition of wellness.
- Wellness is more than an absence of disease.
- When we change our lifestyle, we change our risk of illness and death.
- By staying well, we can continue to be active and productive as we age.
- Making wellness a priority would save our country billions of dollars each year.
- You have choices.

Allie S. Gooding, a Cardiology Clinical Nurse Specialist at Mission St. Joseph's Health System in Asheville, North Carolina, says that "Wellness is not simply the absence of illness, but a life-style which involves self-responsibility, nutritional awareness, physical fitness, stress management, and environmental sensitivity."

As defined by the World Health Organization, "Health is not merely the absence of disease, but a state of complete physical, mental, and social well-being."

The WHO definition is widely accepted, but leaves out an important component of wellness: the spiritual. The author feels that wellness is a sense of physical, mental, social, and spiritual integration that allows the individual to obtain his/her full potential, to improve the his/her quality of life, and to live in harmony with the self and the world.

WELLNESS IS MORE THAN THE ABSENCE OF DISEASE.

- You can be free of disease and still be unwell.
- When harmony is missing, one is at "disease" and does not feel well.

WELLNESS ADDS QUALITY TO LIFE.

Think of the most exquisite moment of your life. Were you sitting on top of a high mountain watching a glorious sunrise or sunset? Were you swimming in the ocean on a hot, sunny day? Had you just seen your first child born? Were you moving into a newly built home? Were you in a far away land, drinking wine by candlelight with someone you really loved?

How would you like to have exquisite moments more often in your life?

This is one of the payoffs of being well. Your body allows you to enjoy life at its best when your complete being is functioning as it should.

WELLNESS REDUCES THE RISK OF ILLNESS.

Some of the most common illnesses directly connected to our unhealthy lifestyles are:

- heart disease
- lung disease
- strokes
- high blood pressure
- some forms of cancer
- cirrhosis of the liver
- diabetes
- sexually transmitted diseases
- stress related illnesses

WELLNESS ALLOWS US TO LIVE NOT ONLY LONGER, BUT BETTER.

No one wants to live to be a hundred if they are bed-ridden the last thirty years of their life. Fortunately, getting old does not mean we have to give up our quality of life.

- Dr. Paul Spangler ran a marathon (26.2 miles) at the age of 92.
- Corina Leslie celebrated her 90th birthday in a unique way...by taking a sky dive.
- Claire Willi, at age 99 was still taking dance classes.

GOOD HEALTH EQUALS FINANCIAL SAVINGS.

- It has been estimated that 97% of all health care costs are caused by 50% of Americans.
- Data from the American Medical Association shows that nearly $1 out of every $4 spent on health care is a result of social behavior that could be changed (smoking, drug and alcohol abuse, violence, etc.).
- $22 billion a year alone are spent on problems directly attributable to cigarette smoking and other tobacco products.
- The abuse of alcohol caused 100,00 deaths and cost Americans $85.8 billion dollars in health care costs in 1988.
- The American Heart Association estimated in 1996 that cardiovascular disease would cost Americans $151.3 billion in treatment and disability.
- Motor vehicle accidents result in approximately $69.5 billion health care costs each year.
- Obesity costs Americans over $30 billion a year for weight-loss programs and products.
- A problem drinker costs his or her employer an average of $4,800 to $7,500 each year.
- Approximately 12 million people are injured, and 70,000 die on the job each year in the U. S., costing employers over $60 billion annually.
- Drugs in the workplace cost employers $11.2 billion a year ($8 billion from reduced productivity).

- 93 million work days are lost each year as a result of low back pain (most lower back pain can be prevented through exercise).
- In 1996 alone, over 282 million antibiotic prescriptions, 76 million anti-anxiety + tranquilizer medications, 23 million sleeping pills and sedatives, and 23 million diet drugs were filled for Americans.
- In 1995, the government spent $1.7 billion on prescription drugs under Medicaid (approximately $1,000 for each nursing home patient).
- There are approximately 106,000 deaths from adverse drug reactions each year.
- In 1994, medical products and drugs cost our country $78.6 billion (in 1996, Americans paid $4 billion for headache pain relievers).
- Nonsteroidal anti-inflammatory drugs (such as ibuprofen, aspirin, and naproxen), cause 7,600 deaths, and result in 76,000 hospital visits each year in the U.S.
- By the year 2000, it is estimated that the average American family will spend $14,500 a year on health care costs, almost double what they spent in 1994.

DOES WELLNESS SAVE US MONEY? YES!

WELLNESS IN THE WORKPLACE

- Participants in the Reynolds Electrical & Engineering Company, Inc.'s wellness program had 21% lower health claim costs that were lifestyle-related than nonparticipants.
- Johnson & Johnson's wellness program (LIVE FOR LIFE) resulted in a savings of $378 per employee by decreasing absenteeism and lowering health care expenses.
- AT&T Communications wellness program has changed employees' lifestyles and made them more aware of their health. They have predicted that if lifestyle changes continue to improve over the next 10 years, their company will save $72 million by reducing heart attack risks, and $15 million by reducing the cancer rate.
- General Mills had a 19% reduction in absenteeism by participants in its employee fitness program, while absenteeism by non-participants increased by 69%.

- At Steelcase, over a six-year period, employees who participated in the corporate fitness program had 55% lower medical claim costs than employees who did not exercise.
- Union Pacific Railroad, after offering a back care program, had an increase in productivity of 10%, and a decrease in absenteeism of 75%.
- MESA, Inc. credits its wellness program for an estimated yearly savings of $1.6 million dollars in health care costs (for 650 employees).
- Beth Israel Hospital (Boston) used stress management seminars to cut mental health claim costs 22% in a year while cutting employee turnover in half during a five-year period.
- DuPont cut absenteeism 47.5% for participants in its corporate fitness program over a period of 6 years.

WELLNESS IN THE HOME

Staying well will save you lots of money. You don't have to have an employer set up a program for you. You, as an individual, have choices. You can choose good eating habits, regular exercise, not to smoke or drink, to reduce stress in your life, and to buckle up your seat belt when you drive.

You can choose to put smoke detectors in your home, and to make your dwelling more "accident-proof." You can choose a healthy environment and not to use medications unless absolutely necessary. You can choose not to use drugs, and not to take unfair advantage of the health care system. These are important words: YOU CAN CHOOSE.

A REAL-LIFE EXAMPLE OF SOMEONE WHO CHOSE

Linda Humston enrolled in the Executive MBA program at Wake Forest, interrupting her normal lifestyle. Eating "fast food" meals and not having enough time to exercise, Linda gained weight and found she did not feel well. Linda decided to do something about her unhealthy lifestyle. She signed up for a walking/jogging program and a weight loss program, and began walking (gradually building up to 3-5 miles a day, 4-5 days a week). She became more selective about what she ate, and signed up for an aerobic dance class that met 2 days a week. Combining a low-fat eating plan with her exercise program, Linda lost 40 pounds, and says she "feels great!"

"Wellness is a choice. When you decide that being well is really important, you find the time to exercise and eat right."
-- Linda Humston
Former Director, Cardiovascular/Pulmonary Services
Johnson City Medical Center

What Do I Need to Do?

*** Become more knowledgeable about wellness
*** Don't smoke or use other forms of tobacco
*** Exercise daily
*** Eat a low fat, high fiber and high carbohydrate diet
*** Don't add salt to your food
*** Buckle your seat belt
*** Keep stress levels under control
*** Maintain good relationships with those around you
*** Make wise choices

A Thought to Remember

High cholesterol, smoking, high blood pressure, and physical inactivity are the major risk factors that cause strokes and heart disease. All of these risk factors can be changed, or at least modified, through lifestyle changes.

Selected Readings For Chapter 1

1. Benson, Herbert, M. D., and Stuart, Eileen, R. N., C., M. S. . THE WELLNESS BOOK. New York: Simon & Schuster, 1992.
2. Cousins, Norman. ANATOMY OF AN ILLNESS AS PERCEIVED BY THE PATIENT. Toronto: Bantam Books, 1981.

3. Erfurt, John, C., "The Cost-effectiveness of Work-site Wellness Programs for Hypertension Control, Weight Loss and Smoking Cessation," Journal of Occupational Medicine, Vol. 33, No. l, pp. 66-73, Jan. 1991.
4. Fries, James F., et al, "Reducing Health Care Costs by Reducing the Need and Demand for Medical Services," New England Journal of Medicine, 329:321-325, July 29, 1993.
5. Ryan, Regina, and Travis, John. THE WELLNESS WORKBOOK. Berkeley: Ten Speed Press, 1988.
6. THE DOCTORS BOOK OF HOME REMEDIES. By the editors of Prevention Magazine Health Books. Emmaus, Pennsylvania: Rodale Press, 1990.
7. THE WELLNESS ENCYCLOPEDIA. Editors of University of California, Berkeley, Wellness Letter. Boston: Houghton Mifflin Co., 1991.
8. THE WOMEN'S COMPLETE HEALTHBOOK, by the American Medical Women's Association. New York: Delacorte Press, 1995.
9. Tully, Shawn, "American's Healthiest Companies," Fortune, pp. 98-106, June 12, 1995.
10. Vickery, Donald M., and James F. Fries. TAKE CARE OF YOURSELF. Reading, Mass.: Addison-Wesley Publishing Company, Inc., 1990.

INTRODUCTION TO CHAPTER 2

Our bodies are our gardens, to the which our wills are gardeners.
-- Shakespeare

As a former athlete, I have always been awed by the amazing ability of the mind, emotions, and body to operate under the most stressful and demanding circumstances, doing fantastic things at full speed.

We are all aware of the body doing unbelievable things. Recently, I read about a father lifting a car off his child, a 79 year-old woman making her 500th trip up a 6,000 foot peak, and a 90 year-old taking a Bungee jump.

It is truly amazing how our bodies are able to function day after day without our conscious demands. The heart beats approximately 72 times a minute. The lungs take in and expel air. Each cell carries out its own responsibilities, and our blood carries nutrients to the most minute corners of our being...all without conscious thought.

Our bodies basically are our earthsuits that allow us to explore our inner and outer world. It is through our bodies that we enjoy our lives, so It is to our benefit to keep them well. The more we know about our bodies, the more we can appreciate these astonishing beings that give us a unique connection to the world we live in.

CHAPTER 2

THE AWESOME MIND AND BODY

WHAT DO I NEED TO KNOW?

- Our mind and body is connected.
- Healing is a natural occurrence, and would take place more often if we didn't interfere by trying to speed up the process.
- Our spirit operates better when our body is well.
- Good mental and physical habits increase our odds of staying well.
- To go where we want to go, it helps to determine our objectives ahead of time.

So often we think of ourselves in fragmented terms...we think we will feel better if we lose weight...we believe everything will be O.K. if we make more money...we think our self-concept will get a boost if we have plastic surgery.

Sometimes, we even look at our body as being detached from our mind, and our mind as having little connection to our spirit. We may even have a vague sense of our body, mind, and spirit doing its own thing in its own way without any clear-cut connection between the three components of our being.

WE ARE CONNECTED

- The mind is connected to the body.
- The body is connected to the mind.

- The brain is connected to the brain.
- The body is connected to the spirit.
- We are one.

MIND-BODY.

Much research has been done on how our physiological body is affected by our mind. Beyond superficial reactions, such as blushing when embarrassed, and perspiring when scared, our feelings, thought processes, and attitudes can affect the health of our physical body. Research has shown:

- People having certain personality traits are more likely to have certain illnesses.
- Stress and emotions can weaken the immune system.
- The mind can alter the autonomic nervous system (heart rate, blood flow, etc.).

The science of studying the interaction between the mind and the immune system is called **psychoneuroimmunology.** Studies dealing with psychoneuroimmunology are very interesting. For example, some studies have shown that a widower grieving for her husband may have a reduced white blood cell count, making the individual more susceptible to disease.

We also know from research that anger, fright, grief, and other intense emotional feelings have resulted in illness, and even death. It is evident that emotions play a big role in our resistance to disease, and in our recovery rate once we are ill.

Studies have also shown that some individuals are able to control their physiological processes by consciously changing their brain wave patterns. Biofeedback is a simple example of this. Indian yogis and individuals from other eastern cultures have developed their mind-body relationship to a much higher degree than most of us. They can change their heart rate, body temperature, respiration, blood flow, and electrical brain patterns at will.

Social and psychological factors can also affect our health at the physical level. Research on "social support," shows that individuals who have sound and strong relationships with family and friends, live longer than individuals who have weak support systems. A study by Dr. David Spiegel showed that group support allowed women with metastatic breast cancer to live an average of 18 months longer than women who did not participate in group support sessions.

A lack of friends and family ties can affect our health as much as eating poorly or not getting enough exercise.

The brain has tremendous power over the body as demonstrated by:

- hypnosis
- the use of placebos (sugar pills) as medicine
- biofeedback

BODY-MIND.

The body also has power over the mind. As we know, chronic pain can cause depression, as can hormone imbalance. A couple of other examples: a brain tumor can change the thought process, often in bizarre ways, and chemical imbalances can make an individual schizophrenic or paranoid.

On the other hand, very positive things can happen as a result of the body-mind connection. Healthy lifestyles, such as jogging or swimming on a regular basis, can result in chemical changes that act as an antidepressant, relieving anxiety and depression.

BRAIN-BRAIN.

The brain even affects the brain. Some psychochemicals produced in the brain can create psychotic disorders. Also, chemicals produced in the brain during strenuous exercise (endorphins), act as morphine, creating what is commonly called the "runner's high."

BODY-SPIRIT.

The fourth dimension of our connected bodies receives less attention in research, but plays an extremely important role in wellness. This dimension, the spiritual or moral dimension, has been down-played in recent years, which may help explain the increased violence and turbulence in our society.

It is very difficult to define spirituality. To simplify, spirituality in this book will refer to the dynamic nature of the human spirit, which is a result of personal values and beliefs including love, faith, honesty, forgiveness, commitment, and belief in a Higher Being. The spiritual dimension adds hope and optimism to the life of the individual.

Defining one's value system is extremely important to the individual's sense of wellness. When your personal values are in conflict, it may not only result in guilt and other forms of negative emotions, but it can result in actual physical problems. Headaches, ulcers, upset stomach, and diarrhea are not uncommon when an individual is dealing with intense guilt, or a conflict in values.

Life-threatening diseases, such as AIDS, can result from a breakdown in moral and spiritual values.

Internal and external relationships are an important component of spiritual wellness. How the individual relates to the self and to a higher being determines the dynamics of the internal relationship, while attitudes and behaviors toward other people compose external relationships. When the individual gets out of harmony with the self, with what the self determines as a higher power, and/or with friends, family, acquaintances, or strangers, there is a negative impact on health.

Having meaning in one's life seems to play a special role in the spiritual health of an individual. When one loses meaning in one's life, the spiritual and physical health of the individual usually declines also.

A strong internal value system can often overcome extreme negative external factors. Having a sense of purpose, challenge, commitment, and a sense of self-responsibility and control over life can often keep an individual healthy even under adverse conditions.

WONDERFUL FACTS ABOUT OUR MINDS AND BODIES

We take so much for granted each day. We wake up, brush our teeth, eat our breakfast, go to work, come home for dinner, and go about our many activities without a second thought of what is really going on--not so much around us--as in us.

We need to become more aware that we are amazing, marvelous, and magnificent creatures. As we go about our external activities, internally 75-100 trillion cells are engaged in their own jobs, keeping our tissues, organs, and systems operating efficiently.

An appreciation of the intricate workings of the body gives a new connotation to wellness. Once we understand what a prized possession we live in, it makes it much easier to strive for good health. The following facts adds emphasis to what wonderful beings we are:

CELLS.

- Most of the 75-100 trillion cells in the body are only microns or millionths of a meter in size.
- Many cells divide about every 10 to 30 hours; some muscle cells only once very few years.
- One brain cell may be connected to as many as 10,000 other brain cells.
- A single drop of blood contains more than 250 million separate blood cells.
- About 25 trillion red blood cells exist in our body. If we were to spread them out, they would cover four tennis courts.
- 3 million red blood cells are produced every second.

THE BRAIN.

- It has been estimated that our brain can store 100 trillion pieces of information.
- The average person only uses about 15 percent of the brain's capacity.

BLOOD VESSELS.

- There are approximately 60,000 miles of blood vessels in the body. If all of our blood vessels were put end to end, they would circle the globe more than twice.

THE HEART.

- The heart weighs about 10 or 11 ounces, yet pumps about 1,800 gallons of blood per day.
- People living to be 100 years old or more have a heart that has beaten 4 billion times, and that will have pumped 600,000 tons of blood.

THE KIDNEYS.

- Our kidneys process about 47.5 gallons of fluid a day, but only about .4 gallon of this is expelled as urine.

THE LUNGS.

- We breathe in and expel 5,000 gallons of air each day.
- Oxygen and carbon dioxide is exchanged through 300 million alveoli (air sacs) in the lungs.
- When relaxed, we take in about a pint of air each time we breathe. During strenuous activity, we take in about five times more air with each breath.
- 13 million cubic feet of air are breathed by the average individual in a lifetime.

THE SKIN.

- The skin on our body weighs about 6-10 pounds.
- It is estimated that a square inch of skin not only contains blood vessels, but approximately 100 oil glands, 65 hairs, numerous nerves, 650 sweat glands, and about 1500 nerve receptors.
- The skin normally expels about a pint of water each day, but it is possible during strenuous activity to lose 3 gallons of fluid in 24 hours through sweating.

HAIR.

- There are 5 million follicles (from which hair grow) in the average body, with about 100,000 of these in the scalp alone.
- The only parts of our body that does not have hair, are the palms of hands, soles of feet, and on our lip.

BONES.

- During each step, the thighbone can withstand an average of 1,200 pounds of pressure per square inch.
- Running puts up to 6 times our total body weight on our lower extremities, sometimes equaling one ton of force.
- The human body has 206 bones (the skull has 28 bones, the spine has 33 bones, and there are 27 bones in each hand).

MUSCLES.

- Muscles give off enough heat to boil a quart of water for an hour.
- The jaw muscles can exert up to 200 pounds of pressure.

THE EAR.

- The canal between the outer and the middle ear contains small hairs and 4,000 wax-producing glands to prevent dust, insects, and other invaders from reaching the hearing mechanism.

THE SENSE OF SMELL.

o It is estimated that our sense of smell is 10,000 times more sensitive than our sense of taste.
o The average person's nose can distinguish about 4,000 different odors; some

individuals can pick out as many as 10,000 different smells.

THE LIVER.

- The largest organ inside our body is the liver (it weighs about 3 pounds).
- The liver can still function even when 90 percent of it is removed.
- At rest, the liver filters 2.5 pints of blood each minute.
- The liver has about 300 billion hepatic cells.

THE INTESTINES.

- The small intestine, if stretched out, is about 18-23 feet long (about 4 times longer than the average person's height).
- One square inch of the small intestine contains 20,000 villi and 10 billion microvilli (these help the intestine process food and liquids).

OTHER INTERESTING THINGS.

- There are 15 million platelets in a drop of blood (platelets make the blood clot after vessel has been cut or injured).
- The average fingernail grows about 1-5 inches a year.
- Our salivary glands secrete approximately 1 1/2 quarts of saliva each day.
- The enamel in your teeth are so tough that it takes half a million revolutions a minute of a dentist's drill to cut through it.

The above is only a fraction of the small miracles that are a part of our body without any conscious thought on our part. When we think about it, the basic skill of walking in itself is a miracle, as many groups of muscles tense and relax in sequence, giving us mobility and balance.

If you really want to be impressed with your body, add to the above that there are about 650 muscles in the human body, and that there are no two fingerprints alike in the world.

We are truly awesome.

THE REAL REASON WE SHOULD STAY WELL

We can talk about the way wellness reduces our risk of heart disease, diabetes, high blood pressure, and we can talk about all of the other health problems that result from poor eating habits, inactivity, too much stress, etc, but that is not the primary reason why we should seek good health.

The primary reason is that the mind and the body can influence the spirit of an individual. For our spirits to soar, our bodies must be able to soar also...or it will drag us down. That's really why balance and wellness in all areas of our life is so important to us. It increases our quality of life tremendously.

I get pleasure out of simple, physical things. I love hiking in the mountains, and jogging across meadows. But my body must be able to go where my mind wants to go...or I will have to forego some of the things that give me pleasure.

All of us have different objectives. I may want to hike into the Grand Canyon and across the Painted Desert (which I do want to!), and you may want to walk up 10 flights of stairs to your office without breathing hard, or you may simply want to lift your grandchild and hug him tight without hurting your back...but regardless of our objectives, it takes a strong, healthy body to allow our mind, emotion, and spirit to enjoy all of the wonder--filled activities available in our lives.

This is not to say that individuals who have physical handicaps or disabilities can not enjoy life, or obtain a high degree of wellness, for they can. Oftentimes, handicaps make us stronger in other areas. However, it does make life easier when we are mobile and our physical bodies are healthy. HEALTHY BODIES ALLOW US TO CHOOSE MOVEMENT TO INCREASE OUR QUALITY OF LIFE.

A REAL-LIFE EXAMPLE OF SOMEONE WHO CHOSE

Denise Gupton has a husband, three children, and a full-time job, but still finds time to exercise. Denise runs 5 miles 4-5 times a week, substituting aerobics when the weather is bad. She recently participated in the March of Dimes WalkAmerica program, pushing her 3-year-old son in a stroller the entire 10 miles. Denise does upper body weight training, and eats a low-fat, meat-free diet, substituting legumes for meats. Denise and her family always incorporate outdoor activities, such as camping, into their vacations.

"To me, wellness is a state of being: to be healthy in mind and body, to live my life fully, enjoy each moment, and be grateful for what I have and what I can become."

-- Denise Gupton
Diabetes Clinician
Caritas Medical Mall

WHAT DO I NEED TO DO?

*** Look at your being (body, mind, spirit) as one unit.
*** Read articles and books on psychology, physiology, sociology, and spirituality. Become knowledgeable about the many facets of the human body and spirit.
*** Get to know yourself better. "Listen" to what your body and intuition tell you.
*** Count your blessings everyday and accent the positive every chance you get
*** Take every opportunity to be mobile, and to strengthen your muscles, even if it only involves walking up a few extra flights of stairs, or lifting light weights.

A THOUGHT TO REMEMBER

Every individual is uniquely different. No one else in the world is quite like you, nor can they contribute to the world in the exact way you can. If you allow your body, mind, and spirit to operate as a unit, your life will flow much smoother, and you will find life much more pleasurable.

SELECTED READINGS FOR CHAPTER 2

1. Benson, Herbert. THE MIND-BODY EFFECT. New York: Simon and Schuster, 1980.
2. Benson, Herbert. TIMELESS HEALING; THE POWER AND BIOLOGY OF BELIEF. New York: Scribner, 1996.
3. Bortz II, Walter M. DARE TO BE 100. New York: Fireside, 1996.
4. Borysenko, Joan. MINDING THE BODY, MENDING THE MIND. Toronto: Bantam Books, 1988.
5. Chopra, Deepak. AGELESS BODY, TIMELESS MIND. New York: Harmony Books, 1993.
6. Chopra, Deepak. PERFECT HEALTH. New York: Simon and Schuster, 1992.
7. Chopra, Deepak. QUANTUM HEALING; EXPLORING THE FRONTIERS OF MIND/BODY MEDICINE. New York: Bantam Books, 1989.
8. Clark, Etta. GROWING OLD IS NOT FOR SISSIES II: PORTRAITS OF SENIOR ATHLETES. Rohnert Park, California: Pomegranate, 1996.
9. Fossel, Michael. REVERSING HUMAN AGING. New York: William Morrow & Co., 1996.
10. Goleman, Daniel, and Joel Gurin, eds. MIND/BODY MEDICINE; HOW TO USE YOUR MIND FOR BETTER HEALTH. Yonkers, N.Y.: Consumer Reports Books, 1993.
11. Hutschnecker, Arnold. THE WILL TO LIVE. New York: Simon and Schuster, 1983.
12. Khatz, Dr. Ronald, Goldman, Dr. Robert. STOPPING THE CLOCK. New Canaan, Conn.: Keats Publishing Co., 1996.
13. KNOW YOUR BODY; THE ATLAS OF ANATOMY. Edited by Riegert, Ray and Henriques, Leslie, Berkeley, California: Ulysses Press, 1995.
14. Locke, Steven, and Douglas Colligan. THE HEALER WITHIN; THE MEDICINE OF MIND AND BODY. New York: Dutton, 1986.
15. Pelletier, Kenneth R. MIND AS HEALER, MIND AS SLAYER; A HOLISTIC APPROACH TO PREVENTING STRESS DISORDERS. New York: Delacorte Press, 1977.
16. Spiegel, David. LIVING BEYOND LIMITS. New York: Times Books, 1993.
17. Steindl-Rast, David. GRATEFULNESS, THE HEART OF PRAYER; AN APPROACH TO LIFE IN FULLNESS. Paulist Press, 1984.

PART 2

WHAT'S KILLING US?

Poor nutrition, lack of exercise, drinking, smoking, drug abuse, and failure to use seat belts--all activities controllable by the individual--account for more than 50 percent of disease, disability, and death in the United States.

- United Way of America
Strategic Planning Committee
May 24, 1980

Half of all deaths can be traced to ten controllable root causes.
- U.S. Public Health Service

INTRODUCTION TO CHAPTER 3

"Man does not die; he kills himself."
— Seneca

All of us know someone who died before their time. My dad died from a heart attack at the age of 54, and I still see him in my mind as a young man. A friend of mine died in a car accident at the age of 38, and my first boyfriend died of cancer before I graduated from high school. All of these people were too young to die, and they left a deep void in the lives of those they left behind.

Many of us think we are destined to die at a certain time and that there is not anything we can do about it. We are wrong. In many cases, we can make choices that will add years to our lives.

Recently, it was estimated that 1.3 million Americans would die prematurely in a year's time. Prematurely means these 1.3 million Americans died before they should have.

It is sad that every day, Americans die from things they could control if they were just knowledgeable and willing to make different choices.

For example, according to the National Center for Health Statistics, approximately 2,148,000 people in the United States died in 1990. Of those 2,148,000 Americans who died, there were only ten types of illnesses that caused 1,757,216 of the deaths. At least half of those 1,757,216 deaths were avoidable. The same is true today.

Think about that statement...half of all the people in our country who die could prolong their lives by taking more control over their health through responsible choices.

This chapter will zero in on the top ten causes of deaths in adults, and the major risk factors for each of these ten causes of death.

Once you know the facts, it is up to you to make the choices that will keep you alive and well for a longer period of time.

CHAPTER 3

SO WHY ARE OUR AWESOME BODIES DYING YOUNG?

WHAT DO I NEED TO KNOW?

- Many people die years before they should.
- Our lifestyles often determine when we will die.
- By changing our lifestyles, we can often add to our life expectancy and our quality of life.
- We do have choices.

TOP TEN CAUSES OF DEATH FOR ADULTS IN U.S.

The most recent research from The National Center for Health Statistics lists the following top ten causes of death for adults in the United States:

1. Heart Disease
2. Cancer
3. Cerebrovascular Disease (Strokes)
4. Chronic Lung Disease
5. Accidents
6. Pneumonia & Influenza
7. Diabetes

8. HIV Infection (AIDS)
9. Suicide
10. Chronic liver disease

What Causes the Above Deaths?

It is important to remember that death is the end result and may have been caused by something other than what is listed on the death certificate. Even though heart disease may be listed as the cause of death, heart disease may be the result of many things, such as a high fat diet, too little exercise, smoking, and high blood pressure, or it may be caused by a genetic factor.

It is these things (risk factors) that we need to be concerned with since they increase our chance of death. The more risk factors we have, the less chance we have to lead a full, productive life. Unfortunately, some risk factors are caused by things which are totally outside our control, such as heredity, our sex, and our age. However, many risk factors are within our control, and can be prevented, or at least reduced, through our lifestyle choices.

Please keep in mind that the list of risk factors that follow in this chapter is not a complete list, and that some of the risk factors overlap or work in combination with each other. For example, some of the deaths from heart disease may be from poor diet and lack of exercise, while other deaths may result from drug abuse alone. Also, some risk factors listed may be indirect causes of death, but still play a major role in putting the individual at risk.

Major Risk Factors

As you look over the list of risk factors for the ten leading causes of death in the United States, note how many times tobacco, diet, physical inactivity, and alcohol use are mentioned.

According to the U. S. Public Health Service, *tobacco, diet, physical inactivity, and alcohol contribute to more deaths in the United States than any other behavior choices.* Whether we use tobacco, eat right, exercise, or consume alcohol is not dependent on our genes, our gender, or our age. We make the decisions about these behavior habits, and have the opportunity to improve our health and our quality of life when our decisions are good decisions.

If we are to avoid premature death and unnecessary illnesses, we must deal with the things that put us at risk.

Look carefully and thoughtfully at the risk factors to the right of each cause of death on the next few pages. Do any of these risk factors apply to you?

	RISK FACTORS
Number 1: HEART DISEASE	- tobacco use - high fat, high cholesterol diet - lack of exercise - obesity - drug use - high blood pressure - elevated cholesterol levels, and/or poor ratio between HDL and LDL - toxic agents - diabetes - oral contraceptives - stress

Note: A smoker's risk of a heart attack is more than twice that of a non-smoker. Forty-five percent of heart attacks happen to people under age 65, and one in three women 65 years and older has heart disease. About 500,000 women die from heart disease each year – almost twice the number of deaths from cancer. A report by the National Association for Sport and Physical Education showed that 40% of children, ages 5-8, have risk factors for heart disease.

	RISK FACTORS
Number 2: CANCER	- tobacco use - some infectious agents - exposure to carcinogenic agents - high fat, low fiber diet - lack of exercise - obesity - alcohol use - sunlight

- smoked, salt cured, and nitrate cured foods
- estrogen
- radiation
- stress

Note: Some common carcinogenic agents are tobacco smoke, radon, ultraviolet light, and smoked foods. One in three Americans will have cancer. Half of all cancers and cancer deaths could be prevented through a healthier lifestyle (not smoking, good nutrition, and physical activity).

	RISK FACTORS
Number 3:	- tobacco use
STROKES	- diet
	- obesity
	- sodium (for some people)
	- lack of exercise
	- heart disease
	- high blood pressure
	- stress

Note: About 150,000 Americans die from a stroke each year, costing the USA $40.6 billion a year. About 2/3 of the people who have a stroke have high blood pressure (one in every 4 adults in America have high blood pressure). Stroke killed more than 96,000 women in 1995.

	RISK FACTORS
Number 4:	- tobacco use
CHRONIC LUNG	- infections and allergies
DISEASE	- air pollution & other toxic agents
	- stress

Note: In 1994, 69 million workdays were lost because of influenza, 22 million because of the common cold, and 3.4 million because of allergies.

So Why are our Awesome Bodies Dying Young?

Number 5:
ACCIDENTS

RISK FACTORS
- alcohol use
- failure to use lap & seat belts and other protective devices such as restraint seats for children and motorcycle helmets
- tobacco (resulting in burns)
- firearms
- drug use
- failure to install smoke detectors
- stress
- weak muscles

Note: On the day Americans change to daylight-saving time, there is a 7% to 8% increase in traffic accidents because of the one hour loss in sleep. When the clock is switched back to Standard time, accidents decrease 7-8%.

Number 6:
PNEUMONIA AND
INFLUENZA

RISK FACTORS
- tobacco use
- infectious agents
- toxic agents (air pollution, etc.)
- stress

Number 7:
DIABETES

RISK FACTORS
- diet
- obesity
- lack of exercise
- viral illness (may trigger auto-immune response, attacking cells that make insulin)
- ethnic background (Blacks, Hispanics, and American Indians are at higher risk than general population)

Note: Diabetes is not a contagious disease, even though a viral illness may cause type 1 diabetes by affecting the autoimmune response. 16 million Americans suffer from diabetes, and more than 8 out of 10 diabetics die from some form of blood-vessel or heart disease. Approximately 123,000 children and teen-agers in the U. S. have Type 1 diabetes. Diabetes cases have increased sixfold since 1958, partly because Americans have become too fat.

Number 8:
HIV (AIDS)

RISK FACTORS
- unprotected sex
- infected drug needles
- blood transfusion (less likely now because of better screening)
- broken skin or cut when in contact with contaminated body fluid

Note: More than 1 million people died of AIDS in 1995, and about 30.6 million people in the world are infected. As of June 30, 1996, the Centers for disease Control and Prevention had recorded 548,102 cases of AIDS in the United States, and 343,000 of these had died. 16,000 people contract AIDS every day.

Number 9:
SUICIDE

RISK FACTORS
- drug use
- alcohol use
- stress
- availability of a firearm
- conflict in relationships

Note: Men commit suicide 4-7 times as often as women. The 65 and older population commits about 20 percent of all suicides in our country.

Number 10:
CHRONIC LIVER
DISEASE AND
CIRRHOSIS

RISK FACTORS
- drug use
- alcohol abuse
- Pollutants in the air (aerosol, bug + paint sprays, smoke, exhaust fumes, etc.)
- hepatitis viruses
- toxic chemicals (on the skin, in food, in air, such as insecticides)

Note: According to the American Liver foundation, 26,000 Americans die each year from chronic liver disease and cirrhosis. Eliminating alcohol abuse would prevent 75-80% of cirrhosis cases.

OTHER RISK FACTORS

Keep in mind that even though stress may not be listed as a risk factor for all ten causes of death, stress may still play a major role because of its effect on the immune system and on the individual's mental ability to make sound decisions regarding his/her health.

Another risk factor that is difficult to pinpoint or prove by quantitative research is the role of relationships in an individual's life. We do know that support systems and smooth and loving relationships are extremely important in the healing process. We also know that conflict, fear, anger, hate, and many other negative emotions can make an individual sick. Consequently, extreme stress and conflict in relationships must be considered as risk factors and as an obstacle to obtaining good health and a sense of well-being. Other risk factors that may not be well defined are (l) poverty, and (2) lack of access to health care.

Poor people have higher mortality rates for lung cancer, high blood pressure, heart disease, injuries, diabetes mellitus and low birth rates. Poor people also have lower survival rates when they have heart attacks or breast cancer.

Individuals without access to a doctor or a hospital, or without access to screening and preventive services, (whether it is from lack of education, insurance, inability to pay, or the distance they must travel), have a higher risk of death than other individuals.

HOW DO WE PREVENT PREMATURE DEATH, AND IMPROVE OUR QUALITY OF LIFE?

In 1993, an excellent study was done by Dr. Michael McGinnis, Director of the Public Health Service office of Disease Prevention and Health Promotion, and Dr. William H. Foege, a former Center for Disease Control director.

In their study, which was published in the November 10, 1993 issue of the *Journal of the American Medical Association*, Dr. McGinnis and Dr. Foege found that **there are ten controllable root causes for half of all deaths in the United States.** These ten principles are given in Part III, and are so important to your health and well-being, that I would like to encourage you to memorize them and post them in your office, in your home, and in your car.

A Real-Life Example of Someone Who CHOSE

J. H. suffered from high blood pressure and was on medication until she changed her eating habits and became involved in a consistent exercise program. As a result of her commitment to better health, she lost 96 pounds. J. H.'s program consisted of walking 3 miles, several times a week, working out to low impact aerobic tapes at least once a week, riding a stationary bike 5 miles 3-4 times a week, and following a low-fat, low cholesterol diet.

"True success depends on lifetime lifestyle changes and not on temporary fad diets and exercise programs."
-- J. H. R.N., Mission St. Joseph's

What Do I Need To Do?

*** Make a list of your risk factors
*** Think about those risk factors, and what you can do to reduce, or eliminate your risk factors.
*** Start preparing myself mentally to make serious lifestyle changes.

A Thought To Remember

Tobacco, diet, physical inactivity, and alcohol contribute to more deaths in the United States than any other behavior choices.

SELECTED READINGS FOR CHAPTER 3

1. McGinnis, J. Michael, MD, MPP, and Foege, William H., MD, MPH. "Actual Causes of Death in the United States. **Journal of the American Medical Association (JAMA),** November 10, 1993, vol. 270, No. 18, pp. 2207-2212.
2. American Cancer Society. "Choice or Chance: Taking Control."
3. American Cancer Society. "Dietary Fiber to Lower Cancer Risks."
4. American Cancer Society. "Nutrition, Common Sense, And Cancer."
5. American Heart Association. "How To Make Your Heart Last A Lifetime."
6. American Heart Association. "Smoking and Heart Disease."
7. American Heart Association. "What's Your Risk of Heart Attack?"
8. American Lung Association. "About Lungs and Lung Disease."
9. National Safety Council. "Preventing Heart Attacks."
10. THE AMERICAN HEART ASSOCIATION COOKBOOK. New York: Ballantine Books, 1984.
11. THE AMERICAN HEART ASSOCIATIONS'S LOW FAT, LOW CHOLESTEROL COOKBOOK. Editor, Scott M. Grundy. New York: Times Books, 1989.
12. AMERICA'S BEST HOSPITALS. The Editors of U. S. News and World Report. New York: John Wiley & Sons, Inc., 1996.
13. American Institute for Cancer Research (free booklet): "From Around the World: International Menus and Recipes to Lower Cancer Risks." Send self-addressed, business size envelope, stamped with 55 cents postage, to: the American Institute for Cancer Research, Dept. AW, Washington, D. C. 20069.
14. Bailey, Covert. THE NEW FIT OR FAT. Boston: Houghton Mifflin Co., 1991.
15. Bartlett, John G., and Finkbeiner, Ann K. THE GUIDE TO LIVING WITH HIV INFECTION. Baltimore: Johns Hopkins University Press, 1994.
16. Benson, Herbert. RELAXATION RESPONSE. New York: Random House, 1992.
17. Dossey, Larry. HEALING WORDS; THE POWER OF PRAYER AND THE PRACTICE OF MEDICINE. New York: HarperCollins, 1993.
18. Dossey, Larry. PRAYER IS GOOD MEDICINE. San Francisco: Harper, 1996.

19. Drezner, Marc K., and Hoben, Kimberly P. EATING WELL, LIVING WELL WITH OSTEOPOROSIS. New York: Viking, 1996.
20. Fries, James F. ARTHRITIS: A TAKE CARE OF YOURSELF HEALTH GUIDE. Reading, Mass.: Addison-Wesley Publishing Co., 1995.
21. Goor, Ron, Goor, Nancy, and Boyd, Katherine. CHOOSE TO LOSE. Boston: Houghton Mifflin Co., 1990.
22. Guthrie, Diana W., and Guthrie, Richard. THE DIABETES SOURCEBOOK. Chicago: Contemporary Books, 1995.
23. Hauri, Peter, and Linde, Shirley. NO MORE SLEEPLESS NIGHTS. New York: John Riley & Sons, 1991.
24. Hoffman, Mathew, LeGro, William, and Editors of Prevention Magazine Health Books. DISEASE FREE. Emmaus, Pa.: Rodale Press, 1993.
25. JOHNS HOPKINS SYMPTOMS AND REMEDIES; THE COMPLETE HOME MEDICAL REFERENCE. By Johns Hopkins University professors and staff medical writers. New York: Random House, 1995.
26. Klein, Allen. THE HEALING POWER OF HUMOR. Berkeley, California: Ten Speed Press, 1991.
27. KNOW YOUR BODY; THE ATLAS OF ANATOMY. Edited by Ray Riegert and Leslie Henriques. Berkeley, California: Ulysses Press, 1995.
28. Kwiterovich, Peter. BEYOND CHOLESTEROL. Baltimore: Johns Hopkins University Press, 1989.
29. McDougall, John A. THE MCDOUGALL PROGRAM: 12 DAYS TO DYNAMIC HEALTH, New York: Flume Books, 1991.
30. Ornish, Dean. EAT MORE, WEIGH LESS. New York: HarperPerennial, 1993.
31. Ornish, Dean. REVERSING HEART DISEASE. New York: Random House, 1990.
32. Page, Helen Cassidy, Schroeder, John Speer, and Dickson, Tara Coghlin. THE STANFORD LIFE PLAN FOR A HEALTHY HEART. San Francisco: Chronicle Books, 1996.
33. PAIN RELIEF SYSTEM. By editors of Prevention Magazine Health Books. Emmaus, Pa.: Rodale Press, 1992.
34. Pickering, Thomas. GOOD NEWS ABOUT HIGH BLOOD PRESSURE. New York: Simon & Schuster, 1996.
35. Piscatella, Joseph. CHOICES FOR A HEALTHY HEART. New York: Workman Publishing Co., 1987.

36. Piscatella, Joseph. CONTROLLING YOUR FAT TOOTH. New York: Workman Publishing Co., 1991.
37. Piscatella, Joseph. DON'T EAT YOUR HEART OUT COOKBOOK. New York: HarperCollins Publishers, 1993.
38. Ryan, Regina, and Travis, John W. WELLNESS; SMALL CHANGES YOU CAN USE TO MAKE A BIG DIFFERENCE. Berkeley, California: Ten Speed Press, 1991.
39. Sarno, John E. HEALING BACK PAIN. New York: Warner Books, 1991.
40. Sherman, S. E., et al, "Does Exercise Reduce Mortality Rates in the Elderly? Experience from the Framingham Heart Study," **American Heart Journal,** vol. 128, No. 5, pp. 965-72, Nov. 1994.
41. Shephard, R. J., "Exercise and Aging: Extending Independence in Older Adults," **Geriatrics,** vol. 48, No. 5, pp. 61-64, May 1993.
42. THE NEW OUR BODIES, OURSELVES. By the Boston Women's Health Book Collective. New York: Simon & Schuster, 1992.
43. THE DOCTOR'S BOOK OF HOME REMEDIES. Editors of Prevention Magazine Health Books. New York: Bantam, 1991.
44. TOTAL NUTRITION. Edited by Victor Herbert, and Genell J. Subak-Sharpe. New York: St. Martin's Griffin, 1995.
45. Tubesing, Dr. Donald A. KICKING YOUR STRESS HABITS. Dulute, Minn.: Whole Person Associates, 1989.
46. Vickery, Donald M., and Fries, James F., TAKE CARE OF YOURSELF. Reading, Mass.: Addison-Wesley Publishing Co., 1990.
47. White, Timothy P., and Editors of the University of California at Berkeley WellncssLetter. THE WELLNESS GUIDE TO LIFELONG FITNESS. New York: Random House, 1993.

PART 3

HOW DO I IMPROVE MY HEALTH?

"...the health of people is really the foundation upon which all their happiness and all their powers depend."

— Benjamin Disraeli, 1877

CHAPTER 4

THE BIG TEN

These next few pages are the most important pages in this book.

The ten principles covered in this chapter are based on research done by Dr. Michael McGinnis, Director of the Public Health Service Office of Disease Prevention and Health Promotion, and Dr. William H. Foege, a former Center for Disease Control director. (McGinnis, J. Michael, MD, MPP, and Foege, William H., MD,MPH, "Actual Causes of Death in the United States," *Journal of the American Medical Association (JAMA)*, November 10, 1993,Vol. 270, No. 18, pp. 2207-2212.). According to their research, half of all deaths in the United States can be attributed to ten controllable root causes.

These ten controllable root causes are the "Big Ten" of several vital principles that will help you improve your health.

Don't take these principles lightly even though you have probably heard them a million times. Focus on each one of them, and if any, or all of them, are risk factors in your life, determine today that you will begin to do something about it.

KEY PRINCIPLE

1

DO NOT USE TOBACCO

DO NOT USE TOBACCO

* Approximately 400,000 Americans die from tobacco use each year.
* In 1993 alone, cigarette smokers cost the nation an estimated $50 billion dollars, and caused 1 in every 5 deaths from heart disease.
* Mothers who smoke 10 or more cigarettes a day cause 26,000 new asthma cases a year among their children.
* Americans smoke 470 billion cigarettes and 4.6 billion cigars a year.
* Healthcare costs of smokers in the military cost the Pentagon $584 million each year.

WHERE DO I GET HELP?

1. AMC Cancer Information & Counseling Line: 1-800-525-3777.
2. American Association for World Health: (202) 466-5883.
3. American Cancer Society: 1-800-227-2345.
4. Asthma and Allergy Foundation of America: 1-800-7ASTHMA.

5. National Cancer Institute Cancer Information Service: 1-800-4-CANCER.
6. Cancer Research Institute: 1-800-223-7874.
7. Lung Line Information Service: 1-800-222-LUNG.
8. National Center for Tobacco-Free Kids: 1-800-284-KIDS.
9. National Coalition for Cancer Survivorship: (301) 585-2616
10. National Stroke Association: 1-800-STROKES.
11. Your local American Lung Association Office.
12. Call local hospital and ask about smoking cessation classes.
13. American Lung Association: http://www.lungusa.org/index.html
14. HealthFinder Web Site: http://www.healthfinder.gov
15. International Cancer information Center, the National Cancer Institute, and the Office of Cancer Communication: http://cancernet.nci.nih.gov
16. National Cancer Institute (Cancer diagnosis, treatment, and clinical trails): http://cancernet.nci.nih.gov
17. National Cancer Institute database (cancer and its treatment) http://wwwicic.nci.nin.gov

KEY PRINCIPLE

2

DECREASE THE FAT IN YOUR DIET & EAT AT LEAST 5 FRUITS & VEGETABLES EACH DAY

DECREASE THE FAT IN YOUR DIET & EAT AT LEAST 5 FRUITS & VEGETABLES EACH DAY

* Fifty eight million American adults are overweight, and spend $33 billion a year to lose weight.
* At least one-fourth of children in the U. S. are 20%, or more, above their ideal weight.
* Research has shown that diet can cause heart disease, high blood pressure, stroke, diabetes, and cancers of the colon, prostate, and breast.
* It has been estimated that more than 35% of all cancer is caused by diet.
* On the average, each American consumes 63 pounds of fats and oils and 54 gallons of soft drinks each year.

WHERE DO I GET HELP?

1. American Cancer Association: 1-800-227-2345.
2. American Diabetes Association: l-800-232-3472.
3. American Dietetics Association Consumer Nutrition Hotline (Registered Dietitian gives answers to nutrition questions, M-F, 9 a.m.-4 p.m. Central Time. Has recorded messages about nutrition topics M-F, 8 a.m.-8 p.m. Central Time): 1-800-366-1655.
4. American Heart Association National Center: 1-800-AHA-USA1.
5. American Heart Association Stroke Connection: 1-800-553-6321.
6. American Institute for Cancer Research: 1-800-843-8114.
7. FDA Center for Food Safety + Applied Nutrition: 1-800-FDA-4010.
8. Information Center of the National Heart, Lung, and Blood Institute (free materials on fat and cholesterol): (301) 251-1222.
9. Juvenile Diabetes Foundation: 1-800-533-2873, or www.jdfcure.org
10. Preventive Medicine Research Institute (Dean Ornish Program): 1-800-775-PMRI, ext. 221.
11. St. Helena Hospital and Health Center (the McDougall Program): 1-800-358-9195.
12. The Vegetarian Resource Group (information for vegetarians): (410) 366-VEGE.
13. Weight Loss Centers:
14. - Pritkin Longevity Center (Santa Monica, California and Miami Beach, Florida): 1-800-421-9911 and (310) 450-5433.
    - Duke University Diet and Fitness Center (Durham, N. C.): 1-800-362-8446.
    - The Hilton Head Health Institute (Hilton Head, S. C.): 1-800-292-2440 or (803) 785-7292.
    - Green Mountain at Fox Run (Ludlow, Vermont): 1-800-448-8106 or (802) 228-8885.
    - Structure House (Durham, N. C.): 1-800-553-0052 or (919) 688-7379.
15. Call your local Health Department for information.
16. American Heart Association: http://www.amhrt.org
17. American Medical Association's "AMA Health Insight": www.amaassn.org/insight

18. Cooking Light: http://cookinglight.com
19. Food and Drug Administration: http://www.fda.gov
20. Healthfinder Web Site: http://www.healthfinder.gov
21. HealthWorld Online: http://www.healthy.net
22. International Cancer Information Center, the National Cancer Institute, + the Office of Cancer Communications: http://cancernet.nci.nih.gov
23. Mayo Clinic Health Oasis: www.mayo.ivi.com
24. Weight Watchers Interactive: http://www.wwgroup.com/

KEY PRINCIPLE

3

EXERCISE DAILY
(MINIMUM OF 15-30 MINUTES)

EXERCISE DAILY

* The lack of exercise is the 2nd leading cause of death from heart disease in the U. S., and lack of exercise and poor diet together cause at least 300,000 deaths each year in the United States.
* According to the 1996 Surgeon General Report, only 22% of Americans meet the minimum guidelines of 30 minutes of moderate activity most days.
* Exercise can reduce the risk of adult-onset diabetes by one-third, decrease the risk of heart disease 35-55 percent, and reduce the risk of cancer of the colon, breast, the female reproductive system, and the prostate.
* In a study by the Cooper Institute for Aerobics research (Dallas), it was found that fit individuals live longer than unfit individuals even if they had other bad habits such as smoking.

WHERE DO I GO FOR HELP?

1. American Council on Exercise: 1-800-529-8227.
2. American Diabetes Association: 1-800-ADA-DISC.
3. American Heart Association: 1-800-AHA-USA1.
4. American Hiking Society: (703) 255-9304.
5. Arthritis Foundation: 1-800-283-7800.
6. Center for Disease Control & Prevention (Division of Nutrition and Physical Activity): 1-888-CDC-4NRG or 1-888-232-4674 (toll-free).
7. ClubSpa USA (provides free listing of day spas in your area): (201) 865-2065.
8. The International Association of Fitness Professional (information on Personal Trainers): 1-800-999-IDEA.
9. National Handicapped Sports: (301) 217-0960.
10. National Exercise for Life Institute (free brochures on "Exercise and Aging," and "Exercise and Back Pain"): 1-800-358-3636.
11. National Heart, Lung, and Blood Institute (free materials on promoting cardiovascular health): (301) 251-1222.
12. National Women's Heart Disease + Stroke Campaign (American Heart Association): 1-888-684-3278.
13. President's Council on Physical Fitness & Sports: (202) 272-3421.
14. Preventive Medicine Research Institute: (415) 332-2525.
15. Special Olympics: (202) 628-3630.
16. Women's Sports Foundation: 1-800-227-3988.
17. Health Clubs and Fitness Centers.
18. YMCA and/or YWCA.
19. Recreational Centers.
20. Fitness and Swimming Classes at Community Colleges and Universities.
21. Check Out Books and Videos on Exercise at Local Library.
22. Ask the Fitness Trainer: http://lifematters.com/lm/fittrain.html
23. American Heart Association: http://www.amhrt.org
24. Fitness World: http://www.fitnessworld.com/
25. HealthWorld Online: http://www.healthy.net
26. Healthfinder: www.healthfinder.gov
27. Mayo Clinic Health Oasis: www.mayo.ivi.com

KEY PRINCIPLE

4

DON'T MISUSE ALCOHOL

DON'T MISUSE ALCOHOL

* Approximately 100,000 deaths result each year from alcohol abuse, and 18 million people in the U.S. are dependent on alcohol.
* A problem drinker costs his or her employer an average of $4,800-$7,500 per year.
* In 1995 alone, 17,274 individuals died from alcohol-related accidents.
* College athletes drink 78% more than non-athletes.
* One study found that binge drinking may increase chance cancer will spread from initial site to other parts of the body.

WHERE DO I GET HELP?

1. Al-Anon, World Service Office: 1-800-344-2666.
2. Alcohol Abuse Emergency 24-Hour Hotline: 1-800-ALCOHOL.
3. Alcohol and Drug Helpline: 1-800-821-4357.
4. Alcohol Rehab for the Elderly: 1-800-354-7089.
5. Alcoholics Anonymous: (212) 870-3400.

6. American Council on Alcoholism: 1-800-527-5344.
7. American Liver Foundation: 1-800-223-0179
8. Children of Alcoholics Foundation: 1-800-359-COAF.
9. Mothers Against Drunk Drivers (MADD): 1-800-438-6233 (Victim Hotline).
10. National Clearinghouse for Alcohol and Drugs: 1-800-729-6686.
11. National Council on Alcoholism & Drug Dependence Hotline (24 hours): 1-800-475-HOPE, or 1-800-622-2255.
12. National Domestic Violence Hotline (24 hours): 1-800-799-7233.
13. National Safety Council: 1-800-621-7619.
14. Alcohol & Drug Abuse Treatment Centers.
15. Local Church Counseling Group.

KEY PRINCIPLE

5

KEEP PREVENTIVE SHOTS AND VACCINES UP-TO-DATE

KEEP PREVENTIVE SHOTS AND VACCINES UP-TO-DATE

* In 1997, worldwide, 52.2 million people died because of infectious diseases.
* Infections cause 740 million nonfatal illnesses and about 90,000 deaths annually among Americans (not counting HIV virus).
* There has been a 58% increase in deaths from infectious disease in the U. S. in the last 15 years.
* Only 30% of 2-year old Americans are properly immunized.
* 900 million females (1/3 of all females in the world) have TB.

WHERE DO I GET HELP?

1. National Coalition for Adult Immunization & National Foundation for Infectious Disease: (301) 656-0003.
2. National Organization for Rare Disorders: 1-800-999-6673.
3. Your local American Lung Association.

4. Department of Social Services.
5. County Health Department.
6. Local Hospitals.
7. Private Physicians.
8. Employee Health Nurse.
9. Health Clinics.
10. U.S. Department of Health and Human Services (Public Health Services, Centers for Disease Control and Prevention, and National Center for Health Statistics): 1-800-222-2225.
11. U.S. Centers for Disease Control and Prevention (information on 12 vaccine-preventable diseases): 1-800-232-2522 (Mon.-Fri., 8 a.m.-11 p.m. EST). Spanish: 1-800-232-0233

KEY PRINCIPLE

6

AVOID EXPOSURE TO TOXIC SUBSTANCES

AVOID EXPOSURE TO TOXIC SUBSTANCES

* Toxic agents such as pesticides, lead in paint, radon gas, asbestos, solvents, food and water contamination, second hand tobacco smoke, and ultra-violet light and radiation kill more than 60,000 Americans each year.
* Carbon monoxide poisoning was responsible for more than 1,100 deaths in 1994. Synthetic chemicals cause at least 30,000 deaths each year, and exposure to toxic agents at work cause 4% to 10% of all cancer deaths.
* Over 1/3 of the poisoning of children happens in the grandparents' home.

WHERE DO I GET HELP?

1. American Cancer Society:1-800-ACS-2345.
2. American Lung Association (call local office).
3. Asthma and Allergy Foundation of America: 1-800-7ASTHMA.

4. Chemical Transportation Emergency Center Information Line: 1-800-262-8200.
5. Emergency Planning and Community Right-To-Know Hotline: 1-800-535-0202 (9 a.m.-6 p.m. EST).
6. Indoor Air Quality Information Clearinghouse: 1-800-438-4318.
7. National Institute for Occupational Safety and Health: 1-800-356-4674.
8. National Pesticide Telecommunications Network: 1-800-858-7378.
9. Regional Poison Control Center.
10. Safe Drinking Water Hotline: 1-800-426-4791.
11. FDA Center for Food Safety and Applied Nutrition: 1-800-FDA-4010.
12. U.S. Agriculture Department Fish, Meat, & Poultry Complaint Hotline: 1-800-535-4555.
13. Vietnam Veterans Agent Orange Victims, Inc.: 1-800-521-0198.

KEY PRINCIPLE

7

KEEP GUNS SECURE OR GET RID OF THEM

KEEP GUNS SECURE OR GET RID OF THEM

* According to 1993 National Center for Health Statistics, more people were killed by firearm death than by motor vehicle accidents in five states and the District of Columbia.
* Adolescents are three times more likely to commit suicide when guns are kept in the home.
* Family members or acquaintances are 43% more likely to be killed by a gun in the home than an intruder.

WHERE DO I GET HELP?

1. Gun Safety Classes (ask local police department about classes in your area).
2. Local Police Department.
3. National Domestic Abuse Hotline: 1-800-799-7233.

KEY PRINCIPLE

8

BE SEXUALLY FAITHFUL TO ONE UNINFECTED PARTNER

BE SEXUALLY FAITHFUL TO ONE UNINFECTED PARTNER

*
* Death from unprotected sex is one of the most rapidly increasing statistics in the top 10 causes of death in the U.S. (approximately 30,000 people in the United States die each year as a result of unprotected sex).
* Every year, 12 million people contract a sexually transmitted disease.
* 22 million people in the world are infected with HIV, while 650,000-900,000 Americans are infected.
* Every year, 40,000 people in the U. S. are infected with HIV.
* It has been estimated that the lifetime cost of treating an HIV person is approximately $119,000. This cost is rising because of new, expensive drugs.

WHERE DO I GO FOR HELP?

1. American Association for World Health: (202) 466-5883.
2. Center for Disease Control STD Hotline: 1-800-227-8922.
3. CDC National Prevention Information Network, National AIDS Clearing House: 1-800-458-5231.
4. CDC National AIDS Hotline: 1-800-342-AIDS 1-800-344-SIDA (Spanish) 1-800-AIDS-TTY (Hearing Impaired)
5. For information on on-going AIDS research: 1-800-TRIALS-A.
6. National Institutes of Health (will refer you to organization that specializes in your illness):(301) 496-5787.
7. National Women's Health Network (information on illnessesthat affect women): (202) 628-7814.
8. Local Hospitals.
9. Local AIDS Support Group.
10. Healthfinder Web Site: http//www.healthfinder.gov
11. Mediconsult: www.mediconsult.com
12. National Institutes of Health: http://www.nih.gov

KEY PRINCIPLE

9

OBEY TRAFFIC LAWS & USE PROTECTIVE DEVICES SUCH AS SEAT BELTS, AIRBAGS, CHILD RESTRAINT SEATS, & CYCLE HELMETS

OBEY TRAFFIC LAWS & USE PROTECTIVE DEVICES SUCH AS SEAT BELTS, AIR-BAGS, CHILD RESTRAINT SEATS, & CYCLE HELMETS

* In 1993, more than 40,000 American died in car accidents (about 5500 were teenagers).
* The number 1 cause of car crashes in American cities is running red lights (2,600 killed in 1996).
* The risk of death in a motor vehicle accident can be reduced by about 45% to 65% simply by wearing lap and shoulder belts.
* Hospital care for people not wearing their seat belt costs $5,000 more than for those buckled up during an accident (cost is $1200 more for motorcyclists who don't wear their helmets).
* In 1994, traffic deaths increased for the first time in five years. Alcohol causes 43% of fatal vehicle deaths in the U. S. (17,000 deaths).

WHERE CAN I GET HELP?

1. 55/Alive Driving Class, American Association of Retired Person (AARP): 1-800-424-2277.
2. Mothers Against Drunk Drivers (MADD Victim Hotline): 1-800-438-6233.
3. National Child Safety Council: 1-800-327-5107.
4. Brain Injury Association's Family Helpline: 1-800-444-6443.
5. U.S. Department of Transportation DOT Auto Safety Hotline: 1-800-424-9393.
6. National Safety Council: 1-800-621-7619.
7. State Highway Patrol.
8. Police Department.

KEY PRINCIPLE

10

DON'T USE ILLEGAL DRUGS

DON'T USE ILLEGAL DRUGS

* 20,000 people in the U. S. die each year from using illegal drugs.
* Approximately 3 million people in our country have serious problems with drugs.
* From 1992-1995, drug use among 12-to-17-year-olds increased 78%.
* According to a National Institute of Drug Abuse Household Survey, 74% of drug-users were employed in 1995, versus 66% in 1991.
* Drugs cause almost 80% of the poisoning deaths in our country.
* 1.7 million Americans were frequent users of

WHERE DO I GET HELP?

1. Drug Help: 1-800-262-2463, or www.drughelp.org
2. National Clearinghouse for Alcohol & Drug Information: 1-800-729-6686.
3. National Council on Alcoholism & Drug Dependence Hotline (24 hours): 1-800-475-HOPE.
4. National Drug and Alcohol Information Treatment & Referral Hotline: 1-800-

662-HELP (English) 1-800-66-AYUDA (Spanish)
5. Narcotics Anonymous: 1-800-896-8896
6. Medic Alert Foundation: 1-800-344-3226.
7. County Health Department.
8. Local Police Department.

CHAPTER 5

OTHER BIG PRINCIPLES

The previous 10 principles in Chapter 4 are the "biggies" in regards to living a long, healthy life, but there are other principles that are extremely important to good health.

This book does not list all the principles of good health by any means, but the principles given in this chapter, combined with the Top Ten Principles in Chapter 4, can greatly increase your chance of living a satisfying and healthy life.

None of us are perfect. None of us will be able to keep all the key principles of good health all the time. However, it is to our advantage to follow as many principles of good health as we can. Even though some principles may be more important than others on a singular basis, varying combinations and the intensity with which we follow them, can change the degree of risk we face.

Take time to read the principles in Chapter 4 and Chapter 5 over and over. Let the words become a part of your thought process, while seriously considering how you can begin to incorporate as many of these principles as possible into your everyday lifestyle. Even making one change could make a difference in your life.

And, don't underestimate the power of the mind to change your life. It has been estimated that 70-80% of visits to the doctor are in the stress-related, mind/body area.

Dr. Herbert Benson, a medical expert in faith and the spiritual aspect of self-healing found that individuals who were taught simple self-healing techniques, had a 34% decrease in trips to the doctor.

The mind is a marvelous part of the body. Use it for positive, and permanent, lifestyle changes.

KEY PRINCIPLE

11

LEARN TO DEAL WITH STRESS

LEARN TO DEAL WITH STRESS

* According to a 1993 U. S. Public Health Survey, 70-80% of visits to the doctor by Americans were stress-related illnesses.
* Chronic psychological stress may increase your risk of sudden cardiac death by six times.
* Emotional stress may cause 40% of all cardiac arrest deaths.
* 61% of workers are less productive, 55% are frequently ill, and 59% want to quit their jobs because of stress.
* The leading cause of lost work hours is stress-related headaches.
* One study found that wounds heal faster when the individual is not stressed-out.

WHERE DO I GET HELP?

1. Alzheimer's Association: 1-800-272-3900.
2. Alzheimer's Disease Education & Referral Center: 1-800-438-4380.
3. American Chronic Pain Association: (916) 632-0922.

Other Big Principles

4. American Institute of Stress: Dept. U, 124 Park Ave., Yonkers, New York 10703.
5. American Massage Therapy Association (call for qualified massage therapist in your area): (708) 864-0123.
6. The American Self-Help Clearinghouse: (201) 625-7101.
7. Anxiety Disorders Association of America: (301) 231-9350.
8. Crisis National Runaway Switchboard (crisis intervention for adolescents), 24 hours: 1-800-621-4000.
9. Grief Recovery Hotline: 1-800-445-4808.
10. Hospicelink (9 a.m.-4 p.m., M-F): 1-800-331-1620.
11. Mind/Body Medical Institute: (617) 632-9530.
12. National Chronic Fatigue Syndrome Association: (816) 931-4777.
13. National Chronic Pain Outreach Association: 1-301-652-4948.
14. National Domestic Violence Hotline (for victims of domestic violence): 1-800-799-SAFE 1-800-787-3224 (for hearing impaired).
15. National Foundation for Depressive Illness: 1-800-248-4344.
16. National Headache Foundation, 1-800-843-2256.
17. National Health Information Center: 1-800-336-4797.
18. National Institute of Mental Health Information Line: 1-800-421-4211.
19. National Mental Health Association: 1-800-969-6642.
20. Panic Disorder Information Line: 1-800-64-PANIC.
21. Stress Reduction Clinic (University of Massachusetts Medical Center): (508) 856-1616.
22. Employee Assistance Program (ask you employer if your company has an EAP).
23. Call YMCA, YWCA, churches, and health clubs about Yoga classes, exercise classes, or other activities they offer for stress reduction. Call local college or university to see if they offer class or workshop in stress reduction.
24. Watch for humor workshops in your local area.

Key Principle

12

Cultivate Strong Relationships

Cultivate Strong Relationships

* Research indicates that social isolation increases the individual's risk of disease.
* Studies also show that people who live alone have more heart disease than those who live with someone, or with a pet, and that individuals with a strong network of family and friends have a longer life span than people without a strong social support system.
* Divorced individuals have more chronic medical problems and complaints, and more deaths from infectious diseases (up to 6 times as many deaths from pneumonia), than married individuals.

Where Do I Get Help?

1. The American Self-Help Clearinghouse: (201) 625-7101.
2. Hugs for Health Foundation: (714) 832-HUGS.
3. National Mental Health Association: 1-800-969-6642.
4. National Runaway Switchboard: 1-800-621-4000.

5. National Self-Help Clearinghouse: (212) 642-2944.
6. ToughLove International, Inc. (self-help program for families and kids): 1-800-333-1069.
7. Join support groups when possible.
8. Select groups that have common interest activities, such as hiking clubs, bowling teams, volunteer organizations, etc.
9. Volunteer at hospitals, homeless shelters, humane shelters, and other places where you will feel needed.
10. Establish strong relationships with family and friends through notes, phone calls, visits, and helpful acts of kindness.
11. Call your local humane shelter and adopt a pet if you live alone.

KEY PRINCIPLE

13

AVOID POVERTY

AVOID POVERTY

* Poor people have higher mortality rates for lung cancer, heart disease, high blood pressure, diabetes mellitus, injuries, neural tube defects, and low birth weights.
* Poverty is the biggest cause for heart disease, pneumonia, and diarrhea among the world's top killers, according to the World Health Organization.
* In 1989, approximately 7.2 million Americans from ages 18-64 had lost all of their teeth, mainly because they could not afford the cost of a dentist, or dental insurance, and/or as a result of poor diet.

WHERE DO I GET HELP?

1. National Resource Center on Homelessness and Mental Illness: 1-800-444-7415 (Press 1).
2. Call Social Services and/or Health Department and ask about free classes on diet, exercise, heart disease, stress management, and other health problems.
3. Call the U. S. Agriculture Department in your area and inquire about free literature and/or free nutrition classes.
4. If housebound, inquire about Meals on Wheels.

5. Check out free health videos and books from your local library.
6. Enroll in health classes at your YMCA, YWCA, churches, community college, etc.
7. Seek out wellness programs on radio and TV.
8. Take every opportunity to educate yourself and to train for a variety of vocations.

KEY PRINCIPLE

14

LIVE WHERE YOU HAVE ACCESS TO HEALTH SERVICES

LIVE WHERE YOU HAVE ACCESS TO HEALTH SERVICES

* Lack of access to primary care (doctor and/or hospital) increases the risk of death, and may lead to complications from a simple illness.
* Americans dying from infectious diseases has increased 58% in the last 15 years. Many of these deaths result from not having access to needed health services.

WHERE DO I GET HELP?

1. Check on health services through friends, physicians, and the Chamber of Commerce before moving into a new area.
2. If you must live in an isolated area, call the closest hospital and university and inquire about educational opportunities/programs and even telemedicine linkups with specialists by satellite.
3. Before you get sick or injured, look for a convenient hospital with a good reputation, and establish a relationship with a doctor.

Other Big Principles

4. If possible, maintain sufficient insurance coverage.
5. Teach your children how to dial 911, how to give your address and other vital information in case of an emergency.
6. Become knowledgeable about HMO's (Health Maintenance Organization), and other health care cost organizations.
7. For a fee, the following will search medical databases and provide report: Medical Information Foundation: 1-800-999-1999. National Network of Libraries of Medicine: 1-800-338-7657. Planetree Health Resource Center: (415) 923-3680.
8. For free brochure, "Helping You Choose the Hospital for You," write to: Joint Commission on Accreditation of Healthcare Organizations, One Renaissance Blvd., Dept. P, Oakbrook Terrace, Ill., 60181.
9. Health A to Z: http://www.healthatoz.com/ (Navigation tool for medicine and health).

KEY PRINCIPLE

15

ACCIDENT-PROOF YOUR LIFE

ACCIDENT-PROOF YOUR LIFE

* Every year, more than 2 million Americans hurt themselves seriously in falls (approximately 30% of Americans 65 and older fall at least once a year).
* Bicycle accidents cause 600,000 severe injuries each year and 16,000 children under 5 fall out of shopping carts every year in America.
* In the last decade, 73,000 Americans have been saved by seat belts, motorcycle helmets, child safety seats, and age-related driving requirements (children under 12 are not safe in front of air bags, even if they are wearing a seat belt).
* Almost one million Americans have lost eyesight from accidents. Wearing protective eyewear could have prevented most of these injuries.
* Preventable accident killed more than 93,300 Americans in 1995. 26,000 people died in the home, and 5,300 died in the workplace.

WHERE DO I GO FOR HELP?

1. Air Ambulance America (Provides long-distance transportation of organs and patients): 1-800-262-8526.
2. American Paralysis Association's Spinal Cord Injury Hotline (9-5 p.m. M-F): 1-800-526-3456.
3. American Sudden Infant Death Syndrome Institute: (8-4:30 p.m. M-F): 1-800-232-SIDS.
4. DOT Auto Safety Hotline: 1-800-424-9393.
5. U.S. Consumer Product Safety Commission: 1-800-638-2772.
6. National Child Safety Council: 1-800-327-5107.
7. National Fire Protection Association: 1-800-344-3555.
8. Brain Injury Association Family Helpline: (9-5 p.m. M-F): 1-800-444-NHIF.
9. National Safety Council: 1-800-621-7619.
10. National Youth Sports Safety Foundation (information on preventing sports injuries in young people): (617) 449-2499.
11. Prevent Blindness America: 1-800-331-2020.
12. Shriners Hospital Referral Line (free orthopedic or burn care for children): 1-800-237-5055.
13. U. S. Coast Guard Customer Infoline (information on boating safety): 1-800-368-5647.
14. U. S. Consumer Products Safety Commission: 1-800-638- 2772, or http://www.cpsc.gov/
15. Know the numbers for your local fire and police department in case of an emergency.
16. Take First Aid Course to prepare for handling accidents, and look up your local Poison Control Center number.

KEY PRINCIPLE

16

DEVELOP A SENSE OF HUMOR

DEVELOP A SENSE OF HUMOR

* Research has shown that laughter can increase resistance to disease, stimulate the internal organs, and increase circulation. It will also help the individual relax, handle stress better, and improve his/her outlook on life.
* Norman Cousins (author of **Anatomy of An Illness**), cured himself of a devastating illness through humor and laughter.
* A sense of humor can help relieve pain.

WHERE DO I GO FOR HELP?

1. The Carmel Institute of Humor: (408) 624-3058.
2. Speakers' Bureau   The HUMOR Project
   110 Spring St.
   Saratoga Springs, NY 12866
   (518) 587-8770
3. Attend a humor workshop or seminar.
4. Check out funny videos.
5. Select humorous television shows to watch.

KEY PRINCIPLE

17

GET SUFFICIENT SLEEP

GET SUFFICIENT SLEEP

* The U.S. Department of Transportation has estimated that lack of sleep contributes to 10,000 fatalities, and 200,000 traffic accidents each year.
* 1 in 4 drivers have fallen asleep while driving, and 1 in 3 Americans say that lack of sleep affects their work.
* Approximately 40 million Americans have chronic sleep disorders, with almost 12 million suffering from apnea.
* Animal studies have shown that lack of sleep can lead to over-eating, and another study showed that sleep apnea may cause weight gain.
* 63 million Americans (1/3 of adult population in U.S.) are at risk for injuries or disease because of lack of sleep.

WHERE DO I GO FOR HELP?

1. American Sleep Apnea Association: (202) 293-3650.
2. National Center on Sleep Disorders Research: Fax (301) 251-1223, or write to: P.O. Box 30105, Bethesda, MD 20824-0105.

3. National Sleep Foundation (free list of sleep disorder centers by geographical location): 202-785-2300.
4. Contact local hospital to see if they have a "sleep lab."
5. Ask your doctor about sleep apnea.
6. Schedule your day to allow sufficient sleep (7-9 hours).

KEY PRINCIPLE

18

EAT LESS

EAT LESS

* There is a 17-55% lower rate of premature death for American women weighing at least 15% less than the average woman of the same height, while one study showed that there was a 20% increase in cancer, and a 70% increase in the risk of death from heart disease in women who gained 22-40 pounds after age 18.
* Research at NASA showed that individuals who stayed lean and active lost only seven percent of their aerobic capacity by age 70, vs. nearly 50 percent loss of aerobic capacity by the average person.
* Research has shown that mice who eat 40% less than other mice have a 100% increase in their life span, and reducing calories by 30% seemed to slow the aging process in monkeys.
* Even small weight gains as an adult leads to a big increase in the risk for diabetes.

WHERE DO I GET HELP?

1. American Cancer Society: 1-800-227-2345.
2. American Diabetes Association: 1-800-232-3472.
3. National Health Information Center: 1-800-336-4797.
4. American Institute for Cancer Research: 1-800-843-8114.
5. If you need help with your eating habits, take a Behavior Modification Class, or join a weight loss group such as Weight Watchers.
6. Go to the reference desk at your local library, and ask if they have anything on new research about diet and nutrition.

KEY PRINCIPLE

19

PET THERAPY

PET THERAPY

* Owning a pet can lower blood pressure, cholesterol, and triglyceride levels, and result in fewer visits to the doctor (just stroking a pet or simply watching fish swim in an aquarium can lower your blood pressure and reduce your heart rate).
* People who own pets have fewer minor health problems overall, and an individual who has a pet is more likely to be alive one year after a heart attack than someone who has a heart attack and does not own an animal.
* Elderly women living alone, and without a pet, have blood pressure 20 points higher than older women who live alone, but have a dog or cat they love.

WHERE DO I GO FOR HELP?

1. Adopt a pet through the humane shelter.
2. Call Real Estate Agents to see if they know of someone who is moving that must give away their pet.
3. Contact your local veterinarian to inquire about animals they are trying to

place for their customers.
4. Look at pet shops, but check out their background for providing healthy pets to customers.
5. Read the ads in your local newspaper.

NOTE: Select a pet carefully. A poor choice (example: a large, energetic dog in a small apartment) can increase the owner's stress, rather than decreasing it.

Other Big Principles

KEY PRINCIPLE

20

ENJOY NATURE

ENJOY NATURE

* Research has shown that natural smells affect our physical and mental health. Some smells make us more productive, some arouse us sexually, some relax us, etc.
* In one study, it was found that heliotropin, vanilla-like smell, decreased feelings of anxiety during MRI testing.
* Our body follows natural rhythms. Relaxing while absorbing the natural rhythms and smells of nature help us deal with stress and anxiety.
* Americans confirm their need to be in touch with nature by making 268.6 million visits to National Parks every year.
* One study found that rural people live longer than people living in the city.

WHERE DO I GO FOR HELP?

1. America the Beautiful Fund (Dedicated to preserving the man made and natural beauty of America): 1-800-522-3557.
2. American Hiking Society: (703) 255-9304.
3. Ferry-Morse Seeds' Garden Help Line (offers advice on growing backyard

edibles): 1-800-283-3400.
4. National Geographic Society: 1-800-NGS-LINE.
5. National Parks and Conservation Association: http://www.npca.org/home/ncpa
6. National Park Service's Parknet (maps, entrance fees to parks, etc.): http://www.nps.gov
7. Natural Resources Defense Council, 40 West 20th St., New York, NY 10011.
8. Rails to Trails Conservancy: (202) 797-5400.
9. Rocky Mountain Elk Foundation: 1-800-843-7633.
10. Sierra Club: (415) 776-2211.
11. Spafinders (helps to locate spas in your area that looks on nature): 1-800-255-7727.
12. Wilderness Inquiry: (612) 379-3858.
13. World Research Foundation (health and environmental issues): (818) 907-5483.
14. World Wildlife Fund: 1-800-634-4444.
15. Take your vacations at natural locations. Enjoy the beach, the mountains, horseback riding, hiking, camping, and other activities in natural surroundings.
16. Find a safe area to hike in, or just "be."
17. Develop a natural spot in your own yard by planting wild flower seeds and fruit trees. Feed the birds and squirrels, and invite wildlife into your yard.
18. Select a park where you feel secure, and that has an abundance of flowers and trees. Eat your lunch there.

KEY PRINCIPLE

21

KEEP YOUR SURROUNDING QUIET & PEACEFUL

KEEP YOUR SURROUNDINGS QUIET AND PEACEFUL

* A study has shown that nature photographs of water in hospital rooms decreases the number of days spent in the hospital, and lessens pain medication.
* At least 10 million Americans have irreversible hearing loss--many individual's hearing has been damaged by loud noises.
* Dangerous noise levels affect 20 million Americans daily.
* Sounds no louder than a vacuum cleaner have been shown to increase the heart rate.

WHERE DO I GO FOR HELP?

1. Better Hearing Institute Hearing Hotline: 1-800-327-9355.
2. Deafness Research Foundation: 1-800-535-3323.
3. National Information Center on Hearing Loss Dial A Hearing Screen Test: 1-800-222-3277 (9 a.m.-5 p.m. EST).
4. Silent retreats: - Abbey of Gethsemane, Trappist, Kentucky

Phone: (502) 549-3117.
- Holy Trinity Monastery, Saint David, Arizona
  Phone: (520) 720-4642.
- Immaculate Heart Center, Santa Barbara, California
  Phone: (805) 969-2474.
- Nada Hermitage, Crestone, Colorado
  Phone: (719) 256-4778.
- Ignatius Retreat Center, Atlanta, Georgia
  Phone: (404) 255-0503.

5. Turn down loud radios, T.V., and don't stay around sources of loud noises.

KEY PRINCIPLE 22

BALANCE YOUR LIFE

BALANCE YOUR LIFE

* According to a 1993 Gallup Poll, 1/3 of Americans would take a 20% pay cut if they could work fewer hours.
* A 1994 Roper poll found that only 27% of Americans were highly satisfied with their jobs--the lowest percentage since polls were started in 1973.
* Burnout caused by a stressful life can weaken the immune system, increase the risk of heart attack, and raise the blood pressure. However, research at the State University of New York, Stony Brook, found that enjoying good experiences, or simple pleasures, can boost the immune system.

WHERE DO I GO FOR HELP?

1. American Holistic Health Association: (714) 779-6152.
2. Plan a weekend at a monastery, convent, or other spiritual center.
3. Eliminate non-vital activities from your life.
4. Take advantage of seminars and workshops on Time Management, Stress Reduction, Simplifying Your Life, etc.

5. Don't buy material things you don't need...give away clothes and house items you don't use.
6. Schedule a quiet time during your day to contemplate and put things into perspective.
7. Talk to people in your church, or other religious leaders, about balancing life.
8. Eliminate the clutter around you.

KEY PRINCIPLE 23

CULTIVATE MORAL & SPIRITUAL WELLNESS

CULTIVATE MORAL AND SPIRITUAL WELLNESS

* A NewsWeek poll found that 58 percent of Americans feel the need for more spiritual growth in their lives.
* One study found that religious individuals had more than three times the chance of being alive 6 months after heart surgery than patients who weren't religious.
* Other research has shown that religion can help people combat cancer, heart disease, and high blood pressure, and may help terminal patients live longer.
* Dr. Herbert Benson, working with the spiritual aspect of healing, found that individuals who were taught simple self-healing techniques, had a 34% decrease in trips to the doctor.
* One study found that when individuals prayed for heart patients, they were less likely to die, even though the patients didn't know they were being prayed for.

WHERE DO I GO FOR HELP?

1. Visit several local churches, and select one that appeals to you (go to Yellow pages for a listing of all churches).
2. Join prayer groups.
3. Read the Bible, or other spiritual material, daily.
4. Take a retreat at a monastery, abbey, convent, or other spiritual center.
5. Go to your library and check out the video tapes, **Healing and the Mind** (Bill Moyers).
6. Browse through a Christian bookstore. Write down a list of books, tapes, and videos that you would like to purchase as you can afford them.

KEY PRINCIPLE

24

SEEK KNOWLEDGE & EDUCATE YOURSELF

SEEK KNOWLEDGE/EDUCATE YOURSELF

* One study found that nearly 30 percent of patients were unable to read basic medical instructions and prescription labels (90 million Americans lack basic literary skills).
* The National Center for Health Statistics found that adults between 25-64 who had not finished high school has a 30 percent higher death rate than those who received their diploma, and had more than a double death rate when compared to those who attended college for at least one year.
* More educated adults have lower death rates for all major causes of death than the less educated adult.

WHERE DO I GO FOR HELP?

1. American Institute for Preventive Medicine (ask about **Healthy Life Guide to Self-Care** and **Being a Wise Health Care Consumer**): 1-800-345-2476.
2. Internet Web Sites:

- American Medical Association: http://www.ama-assn.org
- Centers for Disease Control: http://www.cdc.gov
- Columbia HealthCare: www.columbia.net
- Doctorline: http://doctorline.com
- Environmental Organization Web Directory (good information on nutrition and environment): http://www.webdirectory.com/Health/
- Food and Drug Administration: http://www.fda.gov
- Food and Drug Administration's Office of Women's Health: http://www.fda.gov/womens
- Health Web: http://hsinfo.ghsl.nwu.edu/healthweb
- HealthAtoZ (navigation tool): http://www.healthatoz.com/
- Healthfinder: www.healthfinder.gov
- HealthGate: www.healthgate.com
- HealthWorld (free access to MedLine): http://www.healthy.net
- Medacess: http://www.medacess.com
- Mediconsult: www.midiconsult.com
- Medinfo: http://www.medinfo.org
- Medline (medical research): www.nlm.nih.gov/
- National Cancer Institute database: http://www:icic.nci.nin.gov
- National Health Information Center: http://nhic-nt.health.org
- National Institutes of Health: http://www.nih.gov
- National Library of Medicine: http://www.nlm.nih.gov
- RxList: http://www.rxlist.com
- Thrive: http://pathfinder.com/HLC
- U.S. Department of Health and Human Services: http://www.healthfinder.gov
- Yahoo's Health: http://www.yahoo.com

3. National Organization for Rare Disorders (9-5 p.m. M-F): 1-800-999-NORD.
4. For a fee, following will search Medical databases and provide a report:
    - Medical Information Service: 1-800-999-1999.
    - National Network of Libraries of Medicine (refers you to a medical library in your area): 1-800-338-7657.
    - Planetree Health Resource Center: (415) 923-3680.
5. Call local community college or library and ask about basic reading and writing classes.

6. Read every opportunity you have, and take advantage of free books, videos, audiotapes, etc. at your local library.
7. Buy a good "Take Care of Yourself" Guidebook.
8. Look for articles on health in the newspaper each day. These will keep you up to date with the latest research.

KEY PRINCIPLE

25

WASH YOUR HANDS

WASH YOUR HANDS

* Hospital infections kill more Americans each year than homicides and car wrecks combined (*Health*, November/December, 1996).
* You infect yourself by touching your nose or mouth or rubbing your eyes when germs are on your hands. Washing your hands often can cut your risk of infection.
* Children washing their hands four or more times during the school day had 24% fewer sick days from colds or flu, and missed 2 as many days because of stomach illnesses.
* Only 68% of Americans wash their hands after going to the bathroom (74% women and 61% men).
* It has been estimated that bacteria on dirty hands make 40 million Americans sick each year.

WHERE DO I GO FOR HELP?

1. Local Health Department.
2. Talk to your nurse or doctor about how to stop the spread of infections.
3. Buy anti-bacterial liquid soap, and use it often to wash your hands.

Note: Always wash your hands after going to the bathroom, after shaking hands with an ill person, and after touching anything that may have germs on it (doorknob, dirty linen, commode seat or handle, etc.).

PART 4

A CLOSER LOOK AT A HEALTHY LIFE

"This is living, not to live unto oneself alone."
- Menander

INTRODUCTION TO CHAPTERS 6-10

> "No man is an island, entire of itself; every man is a piece of the continent, a part of the main..."
> -John Donne

We are social creatures. Even though we may live alone, we still live in a world where we must interact with other people, with our environment, and with other beings.

When the individual is unable to live peaceably and responsibly with the world around her/him, the individual's psychological, spiritual, and physical problems intensify and multiply. When this conflict is prolonged, the individual's health suffers.

The dis-ease with our surroundings creates disease within our bodies and minds.

Think about the problems in our world today. The tragedies we read about daily involves the inability of people to get along with those around them. The genocide in Bosnia, the bickering between Democrats and Republicans, the drive-by shootings of innocent people, the bombings in Israel, and the bombings of our embassies are all examples of what conflict between people can do not only to the individual, but to a country.

Individuals can not constantly live in conflict, and expect to be healthy. **Good relationships are a key to good living.**

Relationships are so extremely important, not only to each individual, but to the culture and society around us, that the next five chapters concentrate on five areas involving interaction between the individual and his/her internal and external world. Inability to move smoothly between internal and external worlds make it extremely difficult to obtain a healthy, peaceful, and happy life.

These five areas of internal and external relationships are: personal relationships, stress management, sexual responsibility, protecting our environment, and moral and spiritual integrity. Stress Management may seem out of place in this list, but inability to handle stress can result in destructive behavior that affects family, friends, and even strangers.

Individuals who can relate to people, animals, and the environment in a kind, caring, sensitive, giving way, contribute not only to their own well-being, but also help build a healthy society. As John Donne pointed out..."every man is a piece of the continent...a part of the main." Without that understanding, good health is an abstract term beyond our reach.

Chapter 6

Building Positive Relationships

We have become more solitary people. Twenty years ago, one in ten people lived alone; today, one of every four households consist of a person living alone.

One disturbing trend is that almost one of every two people in our country see a member of their family less than once a month.

In a year's time, one in six households move, and almost one out of four baby boomers divorced within 15 years after getting married.

Our technology has made us more mobile and more urban, but in the process, it has taken away from our sense of community, close friendships, and tight family ties. This lack of social support and the decrease in close relationships leaves the individual feeling fragmented, and can greatly affect the individual's mental, physical, and spiritual health.

In primitive times, individuals banded together to fight off wild animals and to gather food for survival. Even though our physical safety no longer depends on being a part of a group, psychologists are finding that we still possess strong psychological needs to be bonded in meaningful ways to others. Although we may not consciously recognize it, we have subtle needs to have long-term attachments and commitments to other human beings, and even to animals and other types of pets. Research has found that a lack of attachment to other beings result in higher rates of physical and mental illness.

THE IMPORTANCE OF HUMAN CONTACT

Many studies have shown that individuals who score low on "social participation" (basic human contacts) are three to five times more likely to die prematurely than those who score high on the test. Social isolation contributes to our poor health and premature death just like high blood pressure, smoking, and lack of exercise does.

One study found that loneliness may impair the immune system and slow down the response of the natural killer cells. It is possible that feeling close to other people decreases some of the stresses of life, allowing the immune system to operate efficiently.

Several studies with cancer patients have emphasized the importance of support groups in the healing process and in dealing with pain and depression, and in some cases, have even shown a longer survival rate by those participating in weekly support group meetings.

Other research has found:

- Parents who care about their children raise healthier adults (a study of 87 Harvard college men found that individuals who felt less loved by their parents, and perceived their parents as being unjust, had a higher risk of illnesses such as heart disease and hypertension by the time they were 55).
- Conflict in marriage can actually make you sick. (One study found that husbands with loving and supportive wives had angina half as often as those without a positive support system).
- Divorced people have more chronic medical conditions and health complaints, as well as higher mortality rates from infectious diseases.
- Divorced men abuse alcohol twice as much as married men.
- Negative things in our lives that increase our feelings of stress (such as doing things with people we dislike), can weaken the immune system, while doing things that give us pleasure can strengthen it.
- Being alone even affects our eating habits. People tend to eat less when they eat alone (eating with two other people increased the amount eaten by 41% in one study).

THE IMPORTANCE OF HUMAN TOUCH

The human touch is far more important than most of us realize. Massage can improve your sleep, reduce pain, relieve anxiety and depression, help premature babies gain weight, and strengthen the immune system (patients with AIDS who got several massages a week had an increase in the number and activity level of the "natural killer-cells" in the immune system which help fight off colds and viruses). Some other things we know about the human touch:

- Full-term infants who were massaged in a study at the University of Miami cried less, were less stressed and depressed, and were more active than those who were rocked.
- Other studies found that massage reduced nausea and anxiety in children undergoing chemotherapy, improved breathing in asthmatics, and decreased depression in children with diabetes.
- Most blindfolded fathers are able to recognize their newborn baby by stroking the backs of babies hands (mothers can also recognize their baby by stroking the cheeks of babies while blindfolded).

HOW CAN I IMPROVE RELATIONSHIPS?

Good relationships are dependent on many things such as trust, caring, respect, and a sense of closeness. Oftentimes, it takes years to build a strong, solid relationship. But there are many things you can do every day that will help you establish good rapport with those around you, that hopefully, over a period of time, will lead to good, strong, lifetime relationships. Here are a few things:

- Hug and touch other people more, but keep touch non-sexual. Be more open to hugs and touch from others.
- Cut down on distractions when with other people (turn off radio, T.V., etc.). One study found that television is left on by 30% of Americans families while they eat dinner.
- Explore possibility of living in a community similar to planned communities in Europe (families own a private townhouse or home and share in common

facilities such as a large dining hall and kitchen, laundry room, workshops, play areas and parks, etc. Houses are usually clustered together with parking of cars limited to the perimeter so space is available to walk, talk, play, and socialize without the hassles of vehicle traffic.

- Make yourself available to neighbors and friends. Undertake activities outside your house so others can see and talk to you (wash car, work in your garden, walk around the block, etc.).
- Give a party and invite all your neighbors.
- Keep in touch with friends and family by notes, phone calls, offering to run errands, taking elderly to grocery shop and appointments, making personal visits, etc.
- Build a social network with one or more friends by planning to get together at least once a week to do things that all of you enjoy (bowl, go to a movie, picnic at the park, walk, sit and discuss topics of common interest, etc.).
- Do at least 3 kind deeds a day, with at least one of them directed toward a stranger (give a compliment, share a good book, leave a flower on the desk of a co-worker, offer to feed the animals while neighbors are on vacation, volunteer at the hospital or for a non-profit organization, take food to a shut-in, visit an elderly person who lives alone).
- Practice listening to other people.
- Remember that everyone is probably struggling with something in their lives. Make an effort to encourage others, and when possible, to help them succeed.
- Avoid conflict when possible.
- Balance your time with others, and allow time for yourself. Even though we are social creatures, there are times when we need to be alone to relax and contemplate. Some experts believe social interaction can go to the extreme, and create "intimacy overload."
- Volunteer to help others less fortunate. There are many groups set up for this purpose; for example, Habitat for Humanity International, which is a worldwide Christian ministry established to help build homes with the poor and homeless (121 Habitat St., Americus, Georgia, 31709-3498. Phone: (912) 924-6935, ext. 551 or 552).

CHAPTER 7

STRESS MANAGEMENT

Over the years, life has gotten harder and more complicated. Consequently, there are very few individuals today who do not feel "stressed out" as a result of job demands, corporate downsizing, family responsibilities, financial problems, violence in our society, and/or conflict in relationships.

Inability to cope with stress is not confined to adults. A Louis Harris & Associates poll found that teenagers are so stressed out by their fear of crime and violence that one in nine (more than 1 in 3 in high-crime neighborhoods) did not go to school at times, or would cut some classes because of fear for their safety. Almost 1 in 3 said they were afraid they would become victims of a drive-by shooting, and 1 in 4 did not feel safe in their own neighborhood.

Our society has become so stressful that stress-related disorders account for approximately 80% of all trips to primary-care physicians according to the American Institute of Stress. Anxiety disorders, the most common type of mental problems, cost us 65 billion dollars a year.

The bombing of the Federal Building in Oklahoma City, the Centennial Olympic Park in Atlanta, the abortion clinic in Alabama, and the U.S. Embassies overseas has taken even more away from Americans' sense of security.

Everyday life as we used to know it, no longer exists. For the first time, Americans are conscious of terrorists on their own soil, oftentimes, their own countrymen. The loss of innocence has brought a new level of stress for the American public. At the same time, it has brought a togetherness and a helpfulness that reinforces the American spirit.

JOB-RELATED STRESS

Stress is especially intense in today's workplace where job security is a thing of the past. It has been estimated that stress accounts for over half of the workdays taken each year by absentee employees, costing American businesses greatly as they pay out about $150 billion each year as a result of job-related stress. One study found that managers who fired someone doubled their risk of a heart attack during the week after the firing.

Some other findings on stress in the workplace:

- Northwestern National Life Insurance Co. found that 55% of workers under high levels of stress were frequently ill versus 18% of workers with low stress levels.
- Individuals in high stress jobs, with little control, have significantly higher blood pressure readings than employees in less stressful positions.
- A report by the National Safe Workplace Institute in 1993 indicated that stress contributed to 110,000 violent episodes in U. S. workplaces, resulting in about 750 deaths, and a cost of $4.2 billion to businesses.
- A Gallup survey found that personal and family problems caused 22% of working women to feel frequent pressure while on the job, resulting in anxiety or fatigue, muscle pain, headaches, and other physical symptoms.
- A Beverly Foundation study showed that workers who looked after elderly relatives had almost twice as much trouble with their weight, and suffered three times as much depression and anxiety as workers free of that responsibility.

SOME OTHER STRESS FACTORS

Although doctors have long suspected that stress can result in heart attacks, recent research with data from the 1994 Los Angeles earthquake proved that sudden stress can cause cardiac arrest (five times more people died that day from heart attacks than on a normal day).

Researchers at the University of Western Ontario found that individuals who respond to stress and annoyances in their life with jumps in their blood pressure develop more deposits and blockages in their arteries than individuals who can relax during everyday stressful events.

Recent research has shown that new mothers who breastfeed their baby have less stress than mothers who bottlefeed their newborn because breastfeeding produces lower levels of stress-related hormones.

Any of us who have been extremely stressed out, and developed the flu, a cold, or become ill in other ways, can attest to the fact that stress lowers the immune system's ability to fight back. Stress from overly strenuous exercise, such as running the marathon, can also depress the immune system.

A study at Ohio State University College of Medicine (Columbus), found that stressed-out caregivers needed nine more days for wounds to heal than individuals who were not stressed.

We should remember that even our animals can suffer ill health from stressful circumstances. A month after being relocated from Canada to a wilderness area in Tennessee and Kentucky, six elk died from "stress-related" illnesses.

WHAT IS STRESS?

There is no one definition of stress, but most people would agree that change, or anything that causes us to make adjustments can create stress. The more adjustments we have to make, the more stressful our lives become. This is why it is not a good idea to make more than one major lifestyle change at a time. Taking a new job, moving to a new location, and getting married in a short period of time would create more stress than most people could handle well.

Some other things to remember about stress:

1. Stress can be good or bad, dependent upon the individual's reaction. Without stress, most of us would be bored, would not be challenged, and would never reach our fullest potential. However, too much ongoing stress can lead to health problems.
2. What is stressful to one person may not be stressful to another person...which points out that it is our **perception** of a situation that determines our stress level. **By changing how our mind perceives a situation, we can change**

our stress level.
3. The key to handling stress is to learn to relax enough that stress is not in an on-going cycle. Giving your body breathing space during, and between, stressful situations allows it to cope sufficiently without hurting one's health.

How Can I Handle Stress Better?

- Try to develop a sense of humor.
- Ask yourself if the thing that is bothering you will make any difference a year down the road, or is it life threatening? If not, quit worrying about it.
- Exercise daily. Exercise serves as an outlet for emotional frustrations, and increases hormones and chemicals that make us feel calmer.
- Be careful what you eat. Food allergies can put added stress on the body. Getting insufficient vitamins and nutrients hamper the body's ability to repair itself.
- Go to a quiet place, close your eyes, and concentrate on your breathing, or go for a short walk, Coordinate your breathing with your steps.
- Use mental imagery. Make a list of the five most beautiful, serene places you have ever been, and imagine yourself there. Or, picture a soft gold light spreading throughout your body, bringing a sense of peace with it.
- Hug and pet your dog or cat. Touching animals can lower the blood pressure.
- Include something relaxing in each day's plan: take a leisurely hot bath, sit on the side of a lake and feed the ducks, work in your garden, take a walk through a beautiful neighborhood.
- Attend a workshop or seminar on Stress Management.
- Organize yourself, and work on only one problem at a time.
- Rid your life of clutter. Simplify by giving away things you do not use or need.
- Confide in a trusted friend or family member. Build a social network that you can lean on when you need help.
- Don't hold grudges. Forgive others and go on with your life.
- Do helpful things for other people. Volunteer at a hospital, a nursing home, or for non-profit groups.
- Spend time in natural surroundings each day. If this is impossible, buy a tape with nature sounds (birds singing, ocean suft coming in and out, waterfalls and streams, etc.).

- Eliminate as many tasks as you can that you dislike. Practice saying "No" to things that disrupt your life.
- Plan ahead. Keep an extra set of keys to the house and car in case you get locked out or lose them.
- Free your mind from trying to remember thousands of details by writing things down. Put all notes in one location so you don't have to search for them.
- Start and end your day by counting your many blessings.
- If you hate doing something, do it first thing in the morning so you can enjoy the rest of your day.
- Take your phone off the hook while eating, taking a bath, or sharing something important with a mate.
- Learn several techniques for relaxing, such as meditation, deep breathing, mental imagery, progressive relaxation, etc. and utilize at least one of these techniques when you feel your stress level going up.
- Get sufficient sleep and rest. The body and mind can not handle stress easily when you are exhausted.
- Allow time each day for some solitude.
- When someone is a jerk, remind yourself that your life is too important to let someone rude ruin your day.
- Send positive thoughts out to strangers. Remember that everyone is dealing with stress in their life.
- Don't try to do everything perfectly. Allow yourself the right to make mistakes.
- Work on being flexible, and let rigid standards go. If you have to choose between doing something pleasurable like going out to dinner, or cleaning a dirty house, choose the dinner. Your house (and dirt) can be cleaned another day.
- Plan a "getaway" spot for weekends and days off that is quiet and restful.
- Take time to stretch several times a day. Stretching can help reduce muscle tension.
- Play some slow, relaxing music, and take a catnap.
- Avoid caffeine, cigarettes, and alcohol.
- Feed yourself positive thoughts before going to sleep.

If none of the above help, and you find you are unable to handle the stress in your life, seek out counseling. Contact your Employee Assistance Program (EAP) at work, or talk to someone in your church, a close friend, or a qualified psychologist or psychiatrist.

CHAPTER 8

SEXUAL RESPONSIBILITY

Sexual contact can result in more than 25 different diseases. It has been estimated that approximately half of all Americans get a sexually transmitted disease (STD) at least one time by the time they reach 30, and that at least 40 million Americans are affected by one or more STD's today. Each year, there are 12 million more new cases of STD's in the United States.

However, most of us immediately think of AIDS when we think of a sexual disease because of the severity of the disease and the lack of a cure. The number of cases and the deaths are staggering. From 1981 to October of 1995, The Center for Disease Control had 501,310 reported Aids cases in the United States. 62 percent, or 311,381 of those individuals had died.

Even though the number of new cases of AIDS is now decreasing, AIDS recently became the leading killer of Americans 25-44 years old, jumping ahead of accidents as the main cause of death for this age group.

AIDS is a sexually transmitted disease (STD), but it will be discussed separately because of its wide reaching impact.

SOME IMPORTANT FACTS ABOUT AIDS:

- It has been estimated that one in every 92 American males 27-39 years old is infected with the AIDS virus and that one in every 250 North American (all ages) has been infected with HIV.
- In 1996, the World Health Organization (WHO) estimated that on a worldwide basis, 1.5 million children and 18.5 million adults were infected with the AIDS virus.
- In 1997, UNAIDS estimated that 16,000 people a day are newly infected,

and over 30 million people in the world have HIV.
- If the present trend continues, an estimated 8 million people will die, and 40 million adults will be infected by the AIDS virus by the year 2000 (in Asia alone, 10 million people will be affected by the AIDS virus by the year 2000).
- In 1995, the medical treatment for each AIDS's patient cost an average of $119,000 a year. The cost of a new drug, saquinavir, which has to be used in combination with other drugs already on the market, will raise this cost even more (a 3-drug protease inhibitor combination on the market could cost $18,000 a year for the drugs alone).
- The Center for AIDS Prevention Studies, at the University of California Medical School in San Francisco, found that HIV-positive men who are depressed die sooner than HIV-positive men who are more positive in their outlook on life, even though both groups were just as ill.
- Some research has indicated that HIV-infected individuals may be helped by exercise, especially by strength-training (weight-lifting allows the body to use protein more efficiently as muscle is built up).
- An individual infected with a STD increases his/her risk of getting HIV two to five times when exposed to HIV.

How Do I Prevent AIDS?

- Do not have unprotected sex.
- Stay with one faithful, uninfected partner.
- Do not share syringes or needles.

For More Information, Call the CDS AIDS Hotline:

1-800-342-AIDS
1-800-344-7432 (Spanish)
1-800-243-7889 (Hearing Impaired)

SOME IMPORTANT FACTS ABOUT OTHER SEXUALLY TRANSMITTED DISEASES:

- STDs falls among the most contagious diseases in the United States (approximately one in every six adults in our country have a STD).
- All STDs are spread during vaginal, oral, or anal sex.
- Some STDs can be passed through body fluids such as blood, vaginal fluids, and semen, while some can be spread when an individual comes into direct contact with infected skin.
- The cure rate for most STDs is high if treated early. (Chlamydia screening can decrease the risk of pelvic inflammatory disease by 50%).
- Sometimes STDs can be hard to diagnose, especially in women, because often the individuals do not have any symptoms or signs of the disease.
- Women are more susceptible to almost all STDs, including AIDS, because secretions from the male are deposited directly into the female's body, and because the female has a larger genital area for germs to invade.
- Women who are sexually active as an adolescent have a higher risk of cervical cancer.
- Having a STD increases the risk of getting the AIDS virus.
- A STD can be passed to the baby of a pregnant woman who is infected.
- You can not get a STD from swimming pools or toilet seats, only through direct sexual contact (oral, vaginal, or anal).
- STD germs live in body fluids (vaginal secretions, semen, and blood), and infect by entering through the mouth, the vagina, an open sore, a cut, or the anus. Some germs, such as herpes or genital warts, can infect by entering the skin of places such as the genitals.

WHAT ARE SOME OF THE MOST COMMON SEXUALLY TRANSMITTED DISEASES (STDS) BESIDES AIDS?

- Genital Herpes (there are about 500,000 new cases of genital herpes each year, and 45 million Americans are believed to be infected).
- Chlamydia (4 million Americans infected each year).
- Trichomoniasis (generally called "trich," with 3 million Americans

infected every year).
- Gonorrhea (1.4 million Americans get "clap" each year).
- Genital warts (750,000 Americans have venereal warts each year),
- Syphilis ("syph" causes about 9,000 Americans to be infected every year).

WHAT ARE SOME OF THE SYMPTOMS OF STDs?

- pain when urinating
- bleeding from the vagina when it is not your period
- glands in the groin swell
- pain in the abdomen, especially during sex
- unusual smell, or excessive discharge from the vagina
- blisters, bumps, rashes, genital sores, or growths that may, or may not, be painful
- soreness, pain, itching, swelling, discomfort, or irritation in or around the rectum or vagina
- aches, chills, and fever
- STD as a result of oral sex could produce symptoms of white patches or sores within the mouth, or redness, soreness, or swelling in the throat.

HOW DO I PREVENT STDs?

- The only way to totally cut your risk of having a STD is to never have sexual contact with another individual, and to never share drug needles.
- You can greatly reduce your risk by (1) having only one partner who is free of STDs, and who does not have sex with anyone else, (2) by using latex condoms, (3) by using spermicides with a condom, and (4) always using a clean needle (use bleach to clean needle if it must be used twice).

WHERE DO I GET INFORMATION ON STDs?

- American Social Health Association HealthLine: 1-800-972-8500

- National AIDS Hotline (24 hours a day): 1-800-342-AIDS
- National AIDS Information Clearninghouse: 1-800-342-5231
- National Herpes Hotline: (919) 361-8488
- National STD Hotline: 1-800-227-8922
- Go to your local health department.
- See your doctor.

CHAPTER 9

LIVING WITH OUR ENVIRONMENT

In 1962, Rachel Carson wrote a book, SILENT SPRING, warning us of the dangers of losing many of our beautiful birds and subspecies if we did not learn to take better care of our environment.

Although many positive changes came about as a result of Ms. Carson's book, the natural world around us is being threatened in many other ways today. Expanding economic development, population growth, improper use of technology, and the encroachment of humans into wildlife areas is putting a tremendous strain on our environment.

In the fall of 1995, 1,500 scientists from over 50 nations presented a Global Biodiversity Assessment in which they pointed out that:

1. Vertebrate animals and flowering plants are becoming extinct at a much faster rate than first thought. The pace at which they are becoming extinct is 50 to 100 times faster than expected.
2. As thousands of animals and plants become extinct, our lives as humans will be greatly affected. Food supplies, water sources, the energy we use, and our medicines could be threatened.

Unfortunately, as our society uses its natural resources, we are abusing nature in ways that may be irreversible. All of us must become more conscious of our stewardship of plants, animals, insects, and the air we breathe.

Our quality of life will deteriorate greatly if we continue to encroach on the natural patterns of life. Each creature or plant that becomes extinct robs us not only of beauty, but of the harmony of a balanced ecological system.

There are some positive signs that we as a nation are beginning to take more responsible action toward our natural environment. An example of this is the flooding of the Grand Canyon by the Bureau of Reclamation in the spring of 1996 to rebuild the beaches and provide new habitats for endangered fish and other wildlife in the canyon area.

WHAT IS WRONG WITH OUR ENVIRONMENT?

- Smoke, dust, and soot (from fuel sources, from burning and plowing agricultural fields, from factories and other industries, and from fireplaces and the burning of wood) can cause lung damage, throat and nose irritation, and bronchitis, as well as premature death.
- Smog from burning jungle forests in Malaysia in 1997 shut down airports and affected people and countries hundreds of miles away.
- Soot pollution alone causes as many as 60,000 deaths in the United States each year (your life span may be shortened by about a year if you live in an area with moderate to heavy sooty air).
- People who live in one of the most polluted U. S. cities are at a 15% to 17% higher risk of dying prematurely than individuals living in one of the cities rated as having the cleanest air.
- In 1997, more tropical forests burned than at any other time in recorded history, destroying wildlife habitats and sending immense pollution into the air.
- Illnesses such as lung cancer, respiratory diseases, and heart disease has been connected to "poor indoor air quality."
- Carbon monoxide poisoning kills approximately 300 Americans every year.
- The increase in breast cancer has been linked to the environment (working in the chemical and petroleum industries especially puts women at higher risk for breast cancer).
- According to a German study, women who have high levels of PCBs in their blood, are more likely to have endometriosis than women without high levels.
- About every hour, a toxic spill or accident is reported in the U. S.
- Research has shown that several of the chemicals commonly used to treat yards can cause health problems in people and animals.
- Groundwater carries pesticides into drinking water sources, and into streams and rivers. PCBs and DDT are often found in fish caught in lakes. Beef cattle and other animals that we eat store dioxin in their fat, and humans can store

- DDT and similar chemicals in their fat.
- In 1997, about 700,000 fish were killed in 3 states by animal waste spills. (Two trillion, 730 million pounds of animal waste is produced every year).
- Water has been contaminated in 9% of all household wells by excessive nitrate.
- Deformed frogs are becoming more frequent because of "something in the water."
- Children living where yards have been sprayed with pesticides (including 2,4-D, carbaryl, and Diazinon), have four times the risk of having cancer of the soft-tissues and muscles.
- The problem with pesticides is so great that The National Academy of Sciences has urged the government to do more to protect children from pesticides (adults are not as sensitive to pesticides as children are).
- Pfiesteria piscicda, a microorganism, strengthened by pollution, has killed over a billion fish on the east coast since 1991.
- Exposure to the herbicide, Agent Orange, (used in the Vietnam war), may put the exposed individual's children at a 2 2 times higher risk of being born with spina bifida.
- Agent Orange exposure also increases the risk of having 3 different types of cancers: non-Hodgkin's disease, Hodgkin's disease, and soft tissue sarcoma. It is possible it may also cause prostate cancer and multiple myeloma, respiratory cancers in the trachea, larynx, and lungs, skin blistering, and acute transient peripheral neuropathy (a neurological disorder).
- Recent research showed that herbicides used on corn contaminated the tap water in 28 out of 29 cities tested that relied on surface water.
- The Environmental Protection Agency is concerned that everyday exposure to low-levels of chemicals in cosmetics, packaging, furniture, linings of metal food cans, paints, and pesticides may cause reproductive or behavioral disorders in Americans. They have asked industry to upgrade their testing of thousands of chemicals put in everyday products used by the consumer.
- Duke University research found that each of the three chemicals given to Persian Gulf war soldiers to protect them from nerve gas and insects have no harmful effects when used alone, but when the three were mixed together, they caused neurological problems in animals. This raises the question of whether the "Gulf War Syndrome" may have resulted from the combination of the three chemicals given to the soldiers.

- Radioactive dust from the accident at the Chernobyl Nuclear Power Plant in 1986 left 8,000-125.000 Russians dead, disabled 10,000-40,000 workers who tried to clean up the facilities, left 1.5 million children at risk of thyroid cancer, and exposed at least 4 million individuals to high levels of radiation.
- A recent study found that individuals who were exposed to the Chernobyl radioactive fallout have genetic changes that are being passed on to their children and their descendants.
- 75,000 Americans were exposed to high level radioactive fallout from nuclear bomb tests in Nevada in the 1950's, increasing their risk of thyroid cancer.
- Plastic and balloons left in water and on beaches can be deadly to marine life. In 1994, volunteers for the Center for Marine Conservation, cleaned 3,000 beaches in the United States, picking up 5.6 million pieces of trash (about 1/4 of the trash were cigarette butts).
- Even nature itself presents many hazards. Lyme disease (tick-borne disease) has affected more than 71,000 Americans, heat waves can cause illness and death, falling barometric pressure can make people moody and irritable, high tide and a full moon increase criminal behavior, and stormy weather can make arthritis and joint stiffness worse.

WHAT ABOUT OUR HOME AND WORK ENVIRONMENT?

Although our air is cleaner than it was 10 years ago because of the 1990 Clean Air Act, indoor air pollution may affect as many as 30 percent of remodeled or new office buildings (one of the most common chemical pollutants is Formaldehyde).

It is possible that breathing air inside a building, such as in our homes or our offices, may create more health problems than being outside in the open air. Radon gas, asbestos, material in furniture, drapery fabrics, carpets, cleaning solvents, paints, and fumes from heating systems and other sources can build up inside buildings where windows are closed. Our emphasis on well-insulated homes to save energy while heating and cooling has virtually eliminated fresh air inside a building, allowing the build-up of unhealthy fumes smells.

Cooling and heating systems can create another problem by spreading bacteria and chemicals through homes and offices. An example of this is the 1976 Legionnaires' disease that was spread through a Philadelphia hotel air conditioning system.

Even though our environment can create some major health problems, it is the chronic and everyday discomfort of allergies that bother most of us. Sinus problems, nose and eye irritations, and asthma affect about 20 percent of Americans.

Even though an individual may not have an allergy, fumes from kerosene heaters and wood stoves, cigarette smoke, and smells from new carpet, furniture, or paint and other irritants can make a person miserable when adequate ventilation is not available.

DEALING WITH ALLERGIES.

About 15 million Americans have allergies. Some individuals are so sensitive to the fumes, vapors, dust mites, molds, and pollens around them that they virtually have to go into isolation from the environment each of us deal with each day.

For example, one lady suffering from environmental illness had to wear only cotton clothes, used cotton sheets for curtains, wore no makeup, limited her eating to only four foods a day, used corn or olive oil on her skin, and cleaned and washed with baking soda in order to cope with her allergies.

If you suffer from allergies, some of the following information might be of use to you:

- Many people are allergic to dust mites which live in rugs, upholstered furniture, and in carpets (500 mites can live in a grain of dust). To get rid of them:
  - keep the temperature in your home or office below 70 degrees and keep humidity below 45 percent (use a de-humidifier if necessary, but clean regularly with bleach and water).
  - use vinyl, hardwood, or tile floors rather than carpet (close to 100,000 dust mites can live on a square yard of carpet, and one research study showed that allergens can accumulate in carpet at a rate of 100 times that on a bare, polished floor).
  - wash bedsheets in hot water (above 130 degrees) at least once a week.
  - use plastic zippered covers on bed mattress and pillows, or use polyester

- pillows that can be washed.
  - run the vent to your dryer outside to keep humidity from building up in your house.
  - use leather sofa and chairs instead of cloth upholstered furniture.
- If you are allergic to your pet, but you can't stand the thought of giving it away:
  - do not let pet into bedroom.
  - if possible, bathe animal once a week.
  - have someone else brush animal daily (outside the home).
  - vacuum or mop floor every couple of days (wipe walls down before vacuuming or mopping floor).
  - change filter in vacuum often.
  - use nose filters when hugging, brushing, or coming into close contact with your pet, (especially if it is a cat or a dog), and when vacuuming.
- Use baking soda to freshen the air if you are allergic to spray air fresheners.
- Do not allow smoking in your house.
- Install clean air conditioner and heat filters regularly.
- Use electricity rather than gas or wood for cooking and heating (one study indicates that children's asthma problems become worse when a gas range is used).
- When mold or mildew is a problem, use mildew-resistant paint rather than wallpaper.
- If you have a water problem in your basement, store things in boxes on shelves rather than on the floor to decrease chance of mold buildup.
- Use exhaust fan in bathroom to prevent buildup of moisture, and clean shower curtain and bathroom fixtures with a bleach solution.
- Be aware that certain items easily collect dust, such as dried or silk flowers, books, draperies, "sit-arounds", etc. When possible, place items in cabinets with glass doors. In place of draperies, use vertical blinds or roller shades that you can dust with a damp cloth.
- Unless you are allergic to pollen, open windows when weather permits.
- Get rid of roaches (leading cause of asthma attacks).
- Check your air conditioner in your car for fungi and bacteria (3% of cars have them in AC unit).

WHAT ELSE CAN I DO?

Everyday, there seems to be more and more things to cope with as a result of new technology. Not only do we have to deal with pesticides on our fruits and vegetables, but we now have genetic engineering of some of our fruits and vegetables, and even plants that can grow and thrive in mercury contaminated soil.

Researchers working on a better soybean accidentally created a product that caused allergic reactions in people who were allergic to the Brazil nut (a gene from the Brazil nut had been added to the soybean to counteract the soybeans deficiency in an important amino acid).

As a consumer, you can do the following things to help avoid health problems:

1. Request that your grocery only stock natural fruits and vegetables, or label plainly which items have been changed genetically.
2. Avoid as much animal fat as possible, since pesticides and other chemicals can be stored in fat.
3. Don't microwave foods in plastic containers since plastic may leak into the food at high temperatures.
4. Don't use pesticides or other chemicals on your lawn.
5. Avoid the use of plastic PVC water and sewer pipes.
6. As much as possible, try not to use chemicals to clean your house.

Chapter 10

Staying Morally and Spiritually Well

Through the centuries, men and women have searched for the meaning of life. This search has taken many forms, but regardless of the path taken, most individuals have found that the meaning of life must take into account the spiritual dimension as well as the physical, social, and emotional aspects of life.

Our physical body can be seen and touched, and even our mind can be defined in ways we can understand, but the search for spiritual truth and values is a difficult one because what we seek is so intangible. Even defining the word "spiritual" is not easy, although most would agree that it refers to the dynamic, moving force which is the core of our life.

Our spiritual search is made even harder because we have to fragment our spirituality as we deal with the separation of church and state, and as we meet family and workplace expectations. However, we can not separate our private life from our professional life, and expect to feel whole. At the same time, we can not separate our spiritual component from our body and mind, and expect to be well.

The urge to find our spiritual place in our world can be described in many ways, such as "finding peace of mind," "saving our souls," or "reaching a higher consciousness," but regardless of how we label it, each of us has a deep yearning to connect with a dimension of our life that is sacred and transforming.

In a 1994 Newsweek Poll, it was found that 58% of Americans felt the need to grow spiritually. Regardless of whether the object of this spiritual growth is called God, Buddha, Global Spirituality, the Cosmic Force, Love, or whatever, most individuals feel empty and unfulfilled without some link to the spiritual. We constantly seek to connect with the seen, and the unseen, world around us.

SPIRITUAL VALUES AND MORALS.

We can not talk about the spiritual side of life and good health without talking about morals (our sense of right and wrong). It is the transgression of our morals, and the resulting feelings of guilt and anger, that create many of our health problems.

LIVING THE MORAL LIFE.

The lack of morals in our society is evident to anyone who has been a victim of crime. In 1994, for the first time in history, our prison population went over the one million mark (more than double the 1984 prison population). In 1997, there was a 5.2% increase in the nation's adult prison population. Juvenile crime is a constant concern (in 1995, murders by young people jumped more than 22 percent), and children involved in criminal behavior are getting younger each year.

Domestic terrorist acts in Oklahoma City and Atlanta, and violent acts by members of militia groups in our own country emphasize that irrational immoral acts are being committed on a scale never known before in America.

But it isn't just crime and violent acts against us that makes our lives more insecure and less well. Sickness can result when our sense of balance is thrown off even by "little things." When a friend lies to us, a stranger trespasses on our land, or our child breaks a promise, our lives lose some of its quality. When enough quality is taken from our lives, our health suffers.

Amazingly, some animals seem to have a sense of right and wrong according to a report given at the American Association for the Advancement of Science. Research with a group of chimpanzees found that the chimps were willing to share their bananas except with chimps who had shown selfish behavior before. Chimps also show sympathy and will console each other after one had been hurt. Another study showed that chimpanzees could also be deceptive and show empathy whether they really felt it or not.

Unfortunately, many of us humans do not have a clear sense of values today because the teaching of values is restricted for fear of offending someone of a different religion or different beliefs. This lack of a value system has harmed our society in many ways, and needs to be addressed in the home, in our educational systems, in the church, and other organizations.

Values, or a sense of morals, does not have to come from a religious perspective, and should not be offensive to anyone interested in the good of society. There are certain codes of conduct and civil behavior that all of us should be able to agree on that would make our society stronger and more enjoyable. For example:

- integrity
- honesty
- cleanliness
- courtesy
- compassion
- tolerance
- loyalty
- helpfulness
- self-discipline
- fairness

It would be very hard for an individual to grow up as a contributing member of society if he/she has never been taught to respect other people and their property, and if he/she does not have a sense of compassion or caring for humans and animals. Criminal activity results when the individual or an individual's property is not valued.

Regardless of our religious background, the search for truth and morality should encourage each of us to be open-minded to all types of knowledge, including the possible existence of a Higher Being in a cosmos that is awesome in its architectural design.

OUR RESPONSIBILITY TO NATURE.

A sense of morality would have to include an awareness and an appreciation of nature, and an acceptance that every living being, regardless of how minute, has the right and a purpose for being here. Science has demonstrated how each and every one of us (animal, humans, insects, plants, air, water, etc.) contribute to the other's well-being.

Killing other creatures for our convenience is as much a moral decision as deciding whether stealing is wrong. All of us need to make a conscious effort to determine whether devices that kill indiscriminately, such as bug lights, are really necessary. Convenience killing may be easy and time- saving for us, but our planet is paying an awful price as we drive into extinction some of the creatures and plants that help balance our overall ecology system. Recognizing the "rightness" of the balance of nature is a necessity, not only to our survival, but to our happiness and our good health. We have never lived alone on this planet; and it is only through the contributions of the many plants, animals, and insects that life can be sustained on earth. It is not enough to accept the philosophy of "live and let live." Morally, we should feel obligated to protect our environment and the beings that inhabit it, even if it means an inconvenience for us.

Social service workers, law enforcement professionals, and animal protection advocates say that individuals who commit violent crimes, and/or abuse children or spouses, usually also exhibit cruelty toward animals. In fact, cruel behavior toward animals should be taken as a warning sign that the individual may be involved in criminal behavior, or is capable of criminal and violent acts in the future.

How Can I Be More Spiritual and Moral?

It is important to remember that morals can be taught and learned, and it is our sense of morality that makes us open to spiritual development. Some things that will help in spiritual growth:

- Learn from men and women of good moral character, such as Billy Graham, Abe Lincoln, Mother Teresa, etc.
- Make a list of good virtues, and determine how you can incorporate them into your life.
- Establish a code of conduct for your life. The Ten Commandments is a good start.
- Read books that talk about morality.
- Determine that every living thing has value, and make a commitment today that you will not kill or hurt something solely for your convenience.

- Take time each day to meditate and contemplate on the good in life.
- Be thankful for your friends, clothing, food, housing, freedom, and everyday conveniences. Cultivate a spirit of thanksgiving, even for little things.
- Pray daily. If you do not believe in prayer, send out positive thoughts to others who are less fortunate than you are.
- Take time each day to be silent. Listen to what may be in you or around you.
- Simplify your life. Get rid of everything you do not use or need.
- Make it a point to give some of your abundance to people who are not as fortunate as you are.
- Establish relationships with individuals and groups who exhibit the traits you consider to be moral and spiritual.
- If you do something you know is wrong, make it right to the best of your ability. Do not be afraid to say "I am sorry," or "I apologize," or "please forgive me."
- Set priorities. Place virtue and morality at the top of the list.
- Do at least one kind deed each day without telling anyone you did it.
- Volunteer to help others through humitarian organizations such as Habitat for Humanity, soup kitchens for the homeless, and Meals on Wheels.
- Do not harbor anger or resentment.

ANGER AND DEPRESSION.

Research has shown that hostility, resentment, and anger puts an individual at high risk for depression and heart disease. One Belgium study found that individuals who kept negative emotions stoically to themselves were four times as likely to have a fatal heart attack than people who expressed their feelings, while research in the states has shown that individuals who suppress anger are more likely to have heart attacks.

Another study showed that even mild depression after a heart attack increased the chance the patient would die from another heart attack within 18 months (mild depression increased the risk by 17%, severe depression by 20%). Other preliminary research has indicated that church-goers are not only depressed less, but are healthier physically.

Individuals who are solidly grounded spiritually are seldom depressed. And a sense of faith in a Higher Being not only allows an individual to feel positive, but it offers hope to the individual who is struggling with the everyday problems of life.

THE ONE GUIDING PRINCIPLE OF MORALITY.

If you need a simple philosophy for living a moral life, the one principle of morality that will cover all situations, is the "Golden Rule" from the Bible: "Do unto others as you would have them do onto you." Nothing makes us more human or moral than treating other people with the respect and kindness we would want them to show toward us.

Whether we are religious people or not, common sense would point to the wisdom of this principle. If you want to see a change in your own life, and in the lives of those around you, apply the Golden Rule in everything you do.

CAN PRAYER HELP US STAY WELL?

Research indicates that prayer can help heal us and help keep us well.

A study in 1988 by Dr. Randolph Byrd showed that patients who were prayed for were 5 times less likely to need antibiotics, 2 times less likely to have congestive heart failure, and had a lower risk of cardiac arrest than patients who were not prayed for.

Other studies have indicated that prayer can help heal wounds, lower high blood pressure, lessen headaches, and lower anxiety.

The interesting thing in these studies is that prayer did not have to be specific to be beneficial, but may consist of a word or a phrase, such as "The Lord is My Shepherd," "Peace," etc.

Ninety-four percent of HMO executives indicated in a 1997 survey that they believe in the healing power of meditation and prayer, and seventy-four percent indicated spirituality could have a favorable impact on healthcare costs. However, they would like more proof before including it in health plans and insurance payments.

PART 5

WHERE DO I GO FROM HERE?

"Let down your buckets where you are."
- Booker T. Washington

INTRODUCTION TO CHAPTERS 11-13

> "The worst boss anyone can have is a bad habit."
> - Monta Crane

We are busy people. We like things to come easy in our busy worlds because we don't have a lot of free time to deal with extra activities, or difficult decisions.

For most people, major change is difficult to deal with. However, change is an important part of life. Change in our lives can be extremely productive and stimulating, and when done in an organized and well-thought out pattern, it can actually make our lives easier over the long-run.

Without change, we become bored and lose our motivation to do the best we can.

Changing bad habits can certainly make our lives better. Incorporating positive lifestyle changes in our everyday routine can cut our risk of illness and disease, can make us more productive, can reduce absenteeism, can improve our self image, can increase our life span, and can save us money.

Chapter 11 has been written to encourage you to make changes in the habits that are detrimental to your quality of life and to your lifespan.

Chapter 12 deals with aging and good health. One in six Americans will be 65 and older by the year 2020. This could place a tremendous burden on our economy if a large percentage of this older population is chronically ill.

Whether we are young or old, good health does not just happen unless the individual has been exceptionally blessed with healthy genes. Good health and a sense of wellness, in most cases, has to be earned through responsible behavior and the development of positive health habits.

If we develop good health habits when we are young, it will certainly make our golden years much easier. It is even possible that some of us can actually be healthier in old age than we were as young people, provided we are willing to recognize, and make, major lifestyle changes where needed.

Fortunately, as you will see in Chapter 12, most of us can remain active, and stay in good health as we age.

A tremendous amount of material has been covered in this book. The author has tried to keep this information simple, but the complexity of staying well has made this difficult at times. Chapter 13, a summary, has been written to be sure the vital points can be picked out easily by the reader.

And, of course, like most writers, I want to have the last word...and have done so... by leaving you a personal note at the end of the book.

Happy, healthy living to you all.

CHAPTER 11

ESTABLISHING A PLAN OF ACTION

WHAT DO I NEED TO KNOW?

- Habits are learned, so we can teach ourselves new habits.
- We don't have to change all of our bad habits at once.
- Establishing goals and a plan is vital to making lifestyle changes.
- Don't let failure worry you. If you persevere long enough, you will succeed.
- Your body will give you signals when something is wrong. Learn to listen to your body.
- Pleasure can make you healthy, or it can make you ill. Be selective in what gives you pleasure.

We can not afford to depend on our doctor, the nurse, or other experts to tell us what is wrong with us. We have innate wisdom built into our own body, and the body is constantly sending out messages to us if we would just listen to it.

The body talks to us in many ways: a high temperature, knee pain, a sore muscle, sensitive joints, swollen glands, rumblings in the stomach, a tickle in the throat, ringing in the ear, shortness of breath, a catch in the side, itching skin, nausea, bruises, a lump in the breast, and even a twitching in the eye are just a few of the signals from the body that something is wrong.

LEARN TO LISTEN TO THE BODY.

If we would take time to become familiar with the body and how it feels when all is well, it would be easier to determine when something feels "different" or "strange." Once we recognize that certain things precede illness (such as a tickle in the throat before a cold, or tight muscles in the neck when we are under too much stress), we can often intervene and head off sickness. For example, taking extra Vitamin C, gargling with salt water, and getting more sleep when the tickle in the throat is first noticed, might prevent having a cold, or the flu. Or it might at least lessen the severity of the cold.

WHY IS MY LIFESTYLE SO IMPORTANT TO MY HEALTH?

The body is a magnificent machine. It can cope with unbelievable things just to survive, but when too many stressors are placed on the body, the body can make us slow down by becoming ill. Usually, the body bounces back after sufficient rest or a change in the diet, but when the body's needs are not met over a long period of time, it

may become chronically ill because it is no longer able to restore itself to a healthy state.

Our lifestyle, or the way we live day after day, greatly affects our body. Junk food, drugs, lack of exercise, too much stress, lack of sleep, smoking, and constant conflicts are just a few lifestyle habits that can drain the body of its ability to bounce back.

To be healthy, we must rid the body, mind, and spirit of things that burden it. This is what we mean by lifestyle changes. We stop doing the negative things that harm our health, and we begin to engage in positive activities that will make us stronger, happier, and healthier.

WHAT DO YOU WANT OUT OF LIFE?

Often the answer to this question changes as our priorities change. Hopefully, one thing you want is to be well. If you are serious about wanting to be healthy so you can enjoy your life for many years to come, then you are at the point where you can make lifestyle changes. Wanting good health is the first step.

WHAT DO YOU REALLY WANT OUT OF LIFE?

We want many things. Sometimes, money is the most important thing to us. For some people, security at home and in the workplace, a college education for the children, or even a week's vacation might top the list of priorities. It is important that you determine what is really important in your life.

Take a sheet of paper and list the ten top priorities in your life. Is good health near the top of your list? If you did not consider good health as one of your top priorities, it will be very difficult for you to make the necessary changes in your life to obtain it. You must *really* want to be to be well before you will be willing to give up the pleasures that make you ill.

THE ROLE OF PLEASURE.

Pleasure plays an important role in our lives. A study by Arthur Stone, Ph.D., State University of New York at Stony Brook, found that illness often followed a decrease in an individual's pleasurable activities, and that the immune system is strengthened by engaging in pleasant events.

We choose many activities because of the pleasure they give us. Running produces the "runners high," a comedy play results in fun and laughter, and a family get-together leaves us with a sense of caring and closeness.

Pleasure can be a very positive part of our lives. The problem is that all pleasure is not good for us. For example, eating chocolate cake and ice cream can leave us with a good feeling; however, over time, the calories and fat content may lead to excess pounds and clogged arteries. Smoking a cigarette after dinner may be extremely pleasurable to some people, but the habit increases the individual's risk of cancer, respiratory illness, and heart disease.

Many people are unable to change their lifestyle habits simply because they can not give up the things that give them pleasure. We are not willing to deprive ourselves of this sense of immediate pleasure even though the long-term effects may be harmful to our health.

One reason it is so difficult to lose weight is that we must give up the pleasurable feelings that come from eating things that taste good to us. It is especially hard for individuals who have no other pleasures except food.

The key to letting the harmful pleasures go is to find other things in our life that will not only give us pleasure, but that will improve our health while making us feel good. For example, instead of over-eating, try substituting:

- laughter
- close friendships
- animal companionship
- exercise
- beautiful surroundings

What Can I Change?

There are some things we can not change:

- our sex
- our age
- our genetic traits
- sometimes our environment

Fortunately, there are many things we can change, or at least have some control over, that will make us healthier and happier:

- our attitude
- our bad habits
- our diet
- our exercise pattern
- our stress level
- our sleep and rest habits
- our use of drugs and alcohol
- our use of cigarettes and tobacco
- our relationships with other people

DECIDING TO MAKE A CHANGE/CHANGES.

What changes would you like to make in your life?

1. Write down everything you would like to change about yourself that would affect your overall health.
2. Place these changes in the order of their importance to you.
3. Think about each of these carefully. Refer back to Chapters 4 and 5 to determine which lifestyle changes would have the maximum affect on your health. Put a star by the most important ones.

YOU DON'T NEED TO CHANGE EVERYTHING AT ONCE.

Even one change in your bad habits could result in better health, especially if it is a high risk habit such as smoking, diet, or lack of exercise. In fact, you don't want to try and change too many things at once. Not only will several changes add stress to your life, but trying to accomplish too much too fast may result in failure, leaving you frustrated and discouraged.

IF YOU COULD ONLY MAKE ONE CHANGE, WHAT WOULD IT BE?

Go back and look at your list. If you had to choose only one lifestyle change from your list, what would it be?

Take that one change, and deal with it one day at a time. It might be helpful to write out a one sentence statement of your commitment, such as "I will eliminate candy bars and carbonated drinks today." Repeat this several times during the day to reinforce your objective for the day.

Whatever change you select, work with it for several months before undertaking other change/changes in your life. You need to have immediate success, and by selecting wisely at the beginning, you can succeed at your first lifestyle change. If you are successful at first, it will make it easier for you to try other changes in the future.

How Can I Be Successful?.

Your chance for success is much better when you plan ahead. There are two key parts to planning:

(1) You must decide what you want to accomplish (establish goals).
(2) You must decide how you are going to do it (plan of action).

Establishing Goals.

The following will help you in setting up your goals:

- Keep it simple (undertake one thing at a time).
- State your goal clearly (write down exactly what you want to accomplish. Example: I want to lose ten pounds).
- Understand why the goal is important to you (I want to lose ten pounds because I am border-line diabetic).

Establishing a Plan.

Good health habits do not just happen. Without a plan of action, there is very little chance you will achieve your goal. To establish a plan of action, do the following:

1. Set a date to start
   - Allow yourself time to prepare for your commitment.
   - Look at your calendar and be sure your start date does not conflict with other events that will make it impossible for you to stick with your plan (for instance, do not start your weight-loss program on the date of your sister's wedding).
2. Break your goal down into small parts that you can handle:
   - If your goal is to lose ten pounds, plan to lose 1-2 pounds a week. Or, if your goal is to exercise 30 minutes a day, start out with 10 minutes a day for the first week to let your body get used to exercise.

3. Remove obstacles
   - Throw away junk food if you are going to diet.
   - Don't socialize with people who try to sabotage your new way of life.
   - Don't watch commercials or read magazines that show people enjoying the negative health habit you are trying to break.
   - Buy the equipment or clothing you need to be successful (shoes built for walking/jogging, comfortable clothes for aerobic exercise, etc.).
4. Plan ahead for difficult situations (when traveling, choose hotels that have fitness facilities, never go grocery shopping when hungry, etc.).
5. Write down a list of positive pleasurable activities you can substitute for the negative pleasures you are giving up (example: a walk around the block instead of smoking after a meal).

THE IMPORTANCE OF POSITIVE MENTAL HABITS.

It takes time to establish new habits. It also takes a new mental outlook. There will be times when you will fall back into your old habits, and if you aren't careful, you will become very negative about the new goals you are trying to accomplish. To maintain a positive attitude, try the following:

- Be aware of words you use (eliminate thoughts such as "I will never be fit," " I have never been able to lose weight," "I can't stop smoking."
- When a negative thought comes into your mind, immediately say "Stop!". Then replace the thought with a positive sentence ("I am going to be physically fit," "I am going to lose my ten pounds," "This time, I am going to stop smoking.").
- Practice relaxation techniques. Learn to use prayer, yoga, meditation, mental imagery, and other techniques to relax and feel more positive about your life.
- Become friends with different parts of your body, and create a spirit of thankfulness for the way they work: take time to "thank" your feet for taking you two miles around the track, "thank" your stomach for digesting your food each day, "thank" your hands for handling delicate tasks so well, etc.
- Mentally see yourself well and healthy. Imagine a screen inside your head, and project pictures of yourself in perfect health on this screen.
- Use mental imagery to strengthen the concept of healing (Carl Simonton,

M.D., had his patients use mental imagery to cure/cope with their cancer).
- Picture a gold, glowing light warming your body, and relaxing you while it kills any germs present in your body.
- Imagine clear, cool water flowing around all of your organs, washing them clean of anything harmful.
- Replace pain with pictures of sunlight bathing the painful area.
- Imagine yourself taking a hose and washing out the inside of your body. Watch the water flush out all the impurities as it drains out your toes.

WHAT IF I FAIL?

The chances are that you will fail. Most smokers fail 4-5 times before finally quitting. Excellent basketball players miss the basket at least half the time, and Babe Ruth struck out 1330 times while hitting 714 home runs.

Failure is a part of life. Failure becomes a problem only when we let failure become our stopping point. We succeed when we continue to persevere while learning from our mistakes. It is that effort of trying one more time that could make the difference in success or failure. So, as the saying goes, "Hang in there," or "If at first you don't succeed, try, try again!"

ONLY PERMANENT LIFESTYLE CHANGES WILL WORK.

You can't look at your goal as being a temporary thing. Losing five pounds for the trip to the beach, or getting fit to play in a tennis tournament, may help you feel and look better for a while, but for the results to be lasting, the lifestyle change has to be approached as a permanent part of your life.

For that reason, you have to set guidelines for yourself that you can live with forever. Unrealistic goals will doom you to failure. So will lack of flexibility. Flexibility will keep you from feeling so deprived, and help you stay with your plan over a long period of time. If you love chocolate, allow yourself a small piece once a week. A small amount of something you love every once in a while will not sabotage your diet unless you are unable to control your appetite when eating certain foods. If chocolate sends you off on a eating binge for weeks, then you may have to ban it totally from your diet.

You may have to change the way you look at things in order to make permanent changes. For example, instead of thinking in terms of dieting, think in terms of good nutrition. You may want to scan some magazines, and cut out a picture of a body you would like to look like. Then paste a photograph of your face on the body you have cut out. Seeing your ideal self will help implant on your sub-conscious what you are aiming for, and how you will "look" when you obtain your goal.

A Real Life Example of Someone who Chose

Tom Forkner has been involved in his own personal health program for many years. He runs 2-3 times a week for 30-60 minutes, rides a stationary, road, or mountain bike twice a week for an hour to an hour and 50 minutes, lifts weights 2-3 times a week for 30 minutes, and is involved in Karate five hours a week. Tom has been an active runner since 1970, and has run two marathons. He has also made gradual improvement in his diet since 1978, eating foods low in fat and cholesterol, and keeping his body fat percentage close to 7 percent since 1978.

"Even though I have a busy schedule, with two children and a full-time job, I have always made my health and fitness a priority."

-- Tom Forkner
Manager
Franklin (N.C.) Health + Fitness Center

What Do I Need To Do?

*** Make a list of needed lifestyle changes
*** Select the one you want to change the most
*** Write down what you want to accomplish (goal), and how you will do it (plan of action).
*** Break the plan down into small segments so you can experience success immediately (lost 2 pounds in one week).
*** Set a start date
*** Celebrate when you accomplish your goal

A Thought To Remember

Good health and a sense of wellness, has to be earned through responsible behavior and the development of permanent, positive health habits.

CHAPTER 12

GROWING OLDER, GETTING HEALTHIER

WHAT DO I NEED TO KNOW?

- We don't have to be sick as we get older.
- We don't have to be weak as we get older.
- We don't have to lose our quality of life as we get older.
- Our older years, in fact, can be better than our younger years.

In the next few years, Americans are going to have to confront age and how it affects our overall society in ways we have never thought about before because:

- Presently, people 65 years and older make up about 12.6 percent of the United States population. By 2030, the number of 65 year olds and older is expected to more than double, and to exceed 70 million.
- From 2010 to 2030, the growth of the older population is expected to increase by 76%.
- The fastest growing part of our population is the 80 year and older group. In 1990, there were 3 million Americans 85 and older – This is expected to more than double by 2020.
- It has been estimated that by 2050, 1 in every 13 Americans may be 80 years of age and older.
The affect of the aging population on our economy can be staggering. According to the U. S. Public Health Service in a report in the *Journal of*

the American Medical Association, the average American who lives to be 76 years old, will experience about 12 years of poor health. This translates to approximately 4,383 sick days.

LIFE EXPECTANCY.

Our population is growing older, and our life expectancy today is higher than ever. For women in our country, the life expectancy at birth is 78.9, and for men it is 72 (the number of individuals age 50-59 is expected to jump 50% by the year 2006). In 1997, it was estimated there were 50,000-60,000 Americans 100 years or older – 3 times the number in 1980. 500,000 Americans are expected to be at least 100 by 2030. This increase in the number of senior citizens is placing a tremendous strain on our health care system.

As we live longer, we must learn to decrease our risks of chronic illness and degenerative diseases or face a catastrophe in our overall health system and our personal lives. Longer life is of very little use if we are chronically ill and bedridden in our later years. Poor health robs us of our enjoyment of life, as well as our savings. In one year alone, Medicare paid out 4.2 billion alone on broken bones and hips suffered by Senior Citizens.

WHAT ARE SOME OF THE HEALTH PROBLEMS OF OLD AGE?

High Blood Pressure, Joint Ailments. A government- funded study by the University of Michigan of Americans, ages 51-61, found 38% have had high blood pressure at some point in their lives, and that 42% have trouble crouching, kneeling, or stooping (joint ailments are the nation's leading cause of disability, afflicting 9 out of every 100 American adults). Another study found that men who have high blood pressure in their mid-life are more likely to have trouble with their memory and thinking process in old age.

Arthritis. It has been estimated that one out of five Americans (60 million) will have some form of arthritis by the year 2020. Women are affected by arthritis more than men (18% versus 12%).

Suicide. A disturbing trend for older people is that suicides by the elderly jumped almost 9% between 1980 and 1992 although they had been declining for four decades (in 1995, it was estimated that about 24,000 elderly Americans 65 or older attempted suicide). Even though 13 percent of the United States' population is 65 and older, this group commits about 20 percent of all suicides in our country. Experts feel that depression (often undiagnosed) causes 90% or more of suicides by seniors, but loneliness, and an inability to deal with chronic illness over a longer lifespan, along with a greater acceptance of suicide by our society, also play a role.

Alzheimer's Disease. Alzheimer's, a degenerative, incurable brain disease, is another health problem most senior citizens fear. The Alzheimer's Association has estimated that 4 million Americans suffer from Alzheimer's disease, with 98% of the deaths from Alzheimer's happening to people over age 65. It has been estimated that 7 million Americans may have Alzheimer's by 2010. The fact that no one is immune to this ravishing disease was brought home to all Americans when former President Ronald Reagan was diagnosed with Alzheimer's.

Osteoporosis. The risk of osteoporosis (bone loss) becomes greater as one gets older, affecting women more often than men. Lack of exercise, insufficient calcium in the diet, smoking, some prescription drugs (those commonly used to treat arthritis and asthma), use of alcohol and/or caffeine, a high-protein diet, some diseases such as cancer or diabetes, and a vitamin D deficiency can all contribute to osteoporosis. 21 million Americans have degenerative osteoporosis.

Other Ways Old Age Affects Us. Old age doesn't just affect the individual. As we age, the problems of poor health affects all of us. It has been estimated that 10 to 20 percent of people who work today are responsible for caring for an aging parent or a relative. But by the year 2020, it has been estimated that one in three Americans will have to look after an elderly parent. In the next 20 years, more than one in every three workers will be 50 or older.

How will this change our lives, especially if our parents are chronically ill? How will families and the workplace be affected by the large percentage of elderly people who will make up our population in the next couple of decades? Will there be enough nursing homes to care for the aging population? How can we maintain quality of life if most of us are old and sick?

An even more important question, how can I as an individual stay healthy as I age?

EXAMPLES OF SENIORS WHO REMAIN WELL AND HEALTHY AS THEY AGE.

The first thing we need to do is to change our mental image of what we can, and can not do, as we age. The following examples should help us re-focus on the fact that we can be healthy, active, and productive even in our 80's and 90's:

- Jack La Lanne, at age 81, still worked out two hours every day at 5 a.m., even when traveling, and at 83, was still leading seniors in exercise.
- Margaret Stevenson, at age 81, hiked six days a week, and in 1993, she made her 602nd five-mile hike up Mount LeConte.
- By 1997, at age 85, Margaret had hiked up Mt LeConte 718 times.
- Claire Willi, at age 99, was still dancing (she attended her first dance class at age 70).
- Cleo Changler, at age 76, competed as a drag racer, and was ranked eighth in the stock car division of the International Hot Rod Association.
- Marguerite Carter, at age 91, was still taking six mile hikes, and teaching an exercise class two days a week.
- George "Banana" Blair, at age 78, performed six days a week on water skis at Cypress Gardens.
- Paul Spangler, at age 94, was still an active marathon runner (he was 77 when he ran his first marathon). His training included running 21 miles a week, swimming half a mile six days a week, and lifting weights three times a week.
- Corina Leslie, at age 90, took a sky dive to celebrate her birthday. At age 91, her exercise routine included stretching 3 times a week, walking about five miles three days a week, golfing twice a week, and even jumping on a trampoline every once in a while.
- Ruth Rothfarb, at age 90, ran her 11th marathon (26.2 miles).
- Former President George Bush parachuted out of an airplane at age 72.
- Helen Klein didn't start running until age 55. Since then, she has run 100 ultramarathons, 49 marathons, and competed in one Ironman. At 73, she had taken part in the Eco-Challenge in Utah, where she rafted, ran, hiked, canoed, mountain biked, rode horseback, and rock-climbed for 9 days on a 370-mile test of endurance.

- Joe Bruno, at age 80, was swimming a mile and half each day.
- Harry Lubar, at age 94, worked out with weights at the Hebrew Rehabilitation Center for Aged in Boston.
- Chuck Yeagen, first man to break the sound barrier, flew a F-15 jet fighter at age 74 to repeat his earlier feat.
- Jacquest Cousteau was still scuba diving at 80 years of age.
- Ben Satz, at 100 years old, began his day with a 90 minute exercise program.
- Jeanne Clament died at age 122 in France. She learned how to fence at 85, still rode her bike at 100, and did a rap co at 121.
- Farrett Weaver, at 99, still volunteers at Fairfield Memorial Hospital.

Research has shown that if an individual will continue to exercise as he or she gets older, that individual can usually be physically active even into their 80's and 90's.

KEEPING OUR MOBILITY, STRENGTH, AND FLEXIBILITY AS WE AGE.

Some research has indicated that only about 1/3 of the decline in aerobic capacity is caused by aging. Two thirds of the decline is a result of inactivity. Older people become chair-bound and bed-bound because lack of exercise has left their muscles weak, not because they have gotten older. It has been estimated that 92% of Americans do not exercise enough to affect their aging process. One study found that exercise resulting in weight loss could help prevent arthritis.

Simply stated, we lose our ability to move because we do not use our muscles:

- Walking, jogging, swimming, riding a bike, playing tennis, etc., increases our ability to engage in strenuous exercise.
- Using our muscles makes our muscles stronger.
- Stretching and bending helps us stay flexible.

The younger we are when we start exercising, the better, but it is never too late to receive the benefits of exercise:

- Several 86-96 year olds at the Hebrew Rehabilitation Center in Boston were put on a weight training program. These elderly individuals lifted weights 3 times a week, for 10-20 minutes, using weights as light as 5 pounds. The seniors more than doubled their strength after 8 weeks, and their ability to climb steps was increased by 28% and their walking speed increased by 12%. Four of the elderly who were on walkers were able to walk with just a cane after their muscles were strengthened, while two of the 90 year-olds were able to walk without their canes, and one man could get out of his chair unaided.
- Frequency of exercise seems to be more important for older people than the intensity of exercise.
- One study found that elderly people who exercised 3 times a week decreased their risk of gastrointestinal hemorrhages by 30%.
- More than 10 million Americans are incontinent (85% of these are women). Exercises that strengthens the pelvic muscles can often improve, and sometimes cure, this problem.
- Some studies have shown that the disease process can be slowed, or even reversed, by smoking cessation and regular exercise.
- About 30% of Americans 65 and older fall at least once a year (over 300,000 older people fracture their hips each year, costing over $10 billion a year in health care costs).
- Exercise reduces the risk of falls for men and women. In one study using Tai Chi, a Chinese martial art consisting of natural, slow, coordinated movements, reduced the risk of falls by elderly people by 48%.
- A study of 60 and 70 year-old men in Finland who continued to lift weights showed that they had the muscle physiology, the muscle fiber size, and the same muscle strength of a 20-year old.
- Research at the University of California at Irvine showed that exercise may help an elderly person's brain to operate more efficiently, possibly because of improved oxygen and blood flow to the brain.
- Another study found that middle-aged men with high blood pressure have more trouble remembering things and thinking when they get old (exercise can often prevent and/or control high blood pressure).
- A Tufts study showed that postmenopausal women who lifted weights two times a week improved their balance and decreased their risk of osteoporosis.

EXERCISE INCREASES LIFE EXPECTANCY.

The following studies should be encouraging to all of us, regardless of our age:

- A study at Stanford University that followed 10,000 men for 30 years found that those who used 2,000 calories a week in aerobic activity extended their life expectancy by 2.5 years.
- Research at Harvard University on 17,321 men for over 20 years found that those who used at least 1,500 calories a week in aerobic activity such as cycling, swimming, walking briskly, or running had a 25% lower death rate than men using up only 150 calories a week through exercise.
- A recent study found that 60, 70, and 80 year old men who walk two miles a day decrease their risk of dying by almost half.
- Research from the Cooper Institute for Aerobic Research (Dallas) showed that becoming fit reduced the risk of death from heart disease by 52%, and death from other causes by 44%.
- The National Institute of Health (Bethesda, Maryland) found that lack of exercise increases an American's risk of a heart attack more than high cholesterol levels.
- One study with women showed that just 30-45 minutes of walking, three times a week, can decrease the risk of heart attack by half for post-menopausal women.

Although most research on exercise has been done with men, women usually obtain the same physiological results from exercise. Even though exercise results are approximately the same, women do live about 7 years longer than men, and they have more chronic health problems such as osteoporosis and arthritis.

DIET CAN ALSO HELP US LIVE LONGER AND HEALTHIER LIVES.

Research with animals has shown that when they are fed a diet where calories have been cut 40-50 percent, they not only age at a slower pace, but they are more active, live longer, have a more responsive immune system, and are at less risk of life-threatening diseases. It has been speculated that the same would be true for humans.

We do know that:

- When adults gain weight, they increase their risk of diabetes.
- Meat-eaters have a 40% higher risk of death from cancer, and a 20% higher risk of death from other causes than vegetarians.
- Women 65 and older can decrease their chance of a hip fracture by drinking less coffee.
- Preliminary research indicates that a diet high in cholesterol and saturated fat increase an elderly person's chance of blindness by 80%.
- A six year Harvard Study of Greeks 70 years and older found that the Mediterranean diet (cereals, breads, legumes, fruits, vegetables, very little meat and dairy products, olive oil but not much butter and other animal fats, and moderate alcohol), not only kept people healthier, but allowed them to live longer.
- One study of middle-aged men found that the risk of stroke could be decreased by 22% if they ate lots of fruits and vegetables.

The number of people 100 years and older has more than doubled since 1980 (four in five centenarians are women). Research at the University of Georgia Gerontology Center of Americans 100 years old and older found that most of them were lean individuals, they took little medication, they ate in moderation although they didn't stick to a low-fat, low- cholesterol diet, none of them were vegetarians, and they mentally were very independent individuals.

STAYING MENTALLY ALERT AS WE AGE.

If you worry about your mental capacity as you age, keep the following in mind:
- George Bernard Shaw, at age 94, wrote a play.
- Strom Thurmond, at age 93, is the oldest person to ever serve in the U. S. Senate. In the spring of 1996, he entered the race for an eighth term because he had "unfinished business" to take care of.
- Winston Churchill's writings, at age 82, was still exceptional and highly

acclaimed pieces of work.
- Grandma Moses, at age 100, was still painting.
- Audrey Stubbart, age 101, was still working full-time as a proofreader and columnist for a daily newspaper.
- Arthur Rubinstein, at age 89, gave a recital in Carnegie Hall.

Some experts feel the mind is just like the rest of the body, you need to use its capabilities or lose your ability to do so. Mental inactivity seems to have more to do with our thinking patterns than aging since the neurons in the brain can make new connections when they are stimulated. Staying socially and intellectually challenged can help the individual stay mentally alert even as the body ages.

Unfortunately, many older people find themselves thrown into an isolated existence when their spouse dies, or when a loss of hearing prevents them from interaction with others. Still, there are ways to continue to challenge the mind even when living alone or when deaf. Reading, putting together puzzles and solving problems, engaging in a hobby, volunteering at a hospital or other organizations, going back to school, exercising at a sports club or spa, or becoming active in a church are just a few things that can help an individual remain active and mentally challenged.

Several research studies have shown that there is very little, or no loss, of memory in older people who stay physically active. One study showed that walking increased an older person's ability to organize and process information.

SOME OTHER THINGS THAT CAN HELP YOUR MIND STAY YOUTHFUL:

- avoid stress.
- stay organized (designate one place to keep your keys, bills, important papers, etc.).
- Concentrate on things you really want to remember.
- Have a notepad handy to write down grocery lists and items you want to recall later.
- Write all appointments on a calendar.
- Avoid drinking alcohol and taking drugs, and other substances that can harm the brain cells.

- Keep distractions and background noise to a minimum.
- Allow enough time that you don't feel rushed to do things, or go places.
- Repeat the names of new people you meet as you talk to them.
- Learn to associate things in visual images. For instance, if you need milk, sugar, and bread when you go to the store, picture the sugar and bread sitting in a tub of milk.
- Get enough sleep. Memory and learning is enhanced when the individual gets sufficient sleep.
- Be curious. Research indicates curiosity can increase your lifespan by 30%.
- Engage in aerobic exercise. Exercise produces chemical changes in the brain that may improve the efficiency of the brain.
- Eat a well-balanced diet, with a variety of nutrients, especially those with complex carbohydrates, fiber, and B-complex vitamins. However, don't overeat. Too much food can affect the alertness of the mind. Drink lots of water.

SOME OTHER THINGS ABOUT AGING.

Research is coming up with new information on aging everyday. For instance, some research has indicated that osteoporosis may be linked to premature graying. And our technology is allowing us to head toward some unbelievable gadgets and inventions that will counteract the aging process. For example, the Food and Drug Administration recently approved our country's first laser for the correction of nearsightedness (70 million Americans are nearsighted), and some doctors believe that someday we will be able to grow replacement body parts, including a human heart.

We should not fear old age. The individual not only has the ability to age gracefully through healthy lifestyle habits, but future scientific and technological advances will help make old age easier to bear.

THE ROLE OF GENES.

At times we need to be reminded that longevity and good health may depend on our genes, and no matter how hard we pursue good lifestyle habits, our good fortune may depend on the biological traits our parents and grandparents have passed down to us.

DISCOUNTING GENES, HOW CAN I STAY HEALTHY AS I GET OLDER?

The following is a summary of this chapter and some additional tips on staying healthy as you grow older:

- Hearing: avoid all loud noises, including loud music.
- Exercise: weight-bearing exercise, such as walking and running, decreases risk of osteoporosis while weight training increases strength and prevents loss of lean body mass. Aerobic exercise helps the body maintain its ability to deliver oxygen to the muscles during physical activity. Regular exercise can help control cholesterol and raise the HDL levels in the blood, decrease the risk of diabetes, lower blood pressure, reduce body fat, improve sleep, and cut the risk of heart disease.
- Blood Pressure: control weight, stay fit, and limit salt in the diet.
- Strong Bones: exercise regularly (especially using weight bearing exercises), get sufficient calcium through the diet or by taking a multi-vitamin/mineral supplements (for most adults, 1,000 milligrams; for post-menopausal women, usually 1,500 milligrams).
- Eat Well: limit cholesterol, fat, and sodium, and eat adequate sources of fiber and carbohydrates (eat 5 or more servings of fruits and vegetables a day).
- Maintain Weight: being overweight can increase your risk of having poor health as you age. Limit fat grams and calories, and exercise regularly.
- Use Safety Cautions: Buckle seat belt, be careful on ladders and around throw rugs. Wait for eyes to adjust when entering dark room, use a sunscreen when outside, etc.
- Be Careful Lifting: Use sound body mechanics when carrying, pushing, or lifting loads to prevent back injuries. Strengthen stomach and leg muscles to

help prevent back strain.
- Health Habits: Start good health habits when you are young because some degenerative conditions start in your teens. Ignore fads, and stick with health habits that have been proven to work. Don't smoke, use tobacco, or abuse drugs. Drink only in moderation.
- Limit Stress: Simplify your life. Learn to breathe deeply, and to relax your muscles when life becomes too stressful.
- Avoid Pesticides and Toxic Chemicals: Wash fruits and vegetables before eating them. Read labels carefully before buying house-cleaning supplies.
- Medical Care: Establish a relationship with a primary-care doctor before you need medical care. Be knowledgeable about health issues, and ask questions about any prescribed medicines. Live in an area where you have access to good medical care.
- Make Friends: Social isolation increases your risk of illness. Establish a network of friends you can interact with and depend on.
- Have a Pet: Research has shown that a pet can be a positive influence on good health. However, poor selection of a pet can be a hassle, and increase stress in your life.
- Contribute to Others: giving to those around you through volunteer work, acts of kindness, and thoughtfulness will not only make your community a better place in which to live, but it will add to your quality of life and to your own good health.
- Seek Pleasure: taking part in activities that are pleasurable can improve your health. Relax and enjoy your life. This is so important to your quality of life that more will be said on this topic in the next paragraph.

Have Fun! None of us want to get to the end of our lives and realize we have not lived well. "Living well" has to include undertaking activities that are fun and pleasurable. Play is such an innate part of life that animals and humans at a young age engage in playful activity. All of us have laughed at puppies crawling over each over and pulling on each other's tails or chasing each over across the yard.

Humans too are born playful. School yards are full of the sounds of children playing. It is only when we get older that we become more serious and less playful as we turn toward making a living and raising a family. Life becomes even more serious as we age and have to face the physical and financial problems of growing older.

However, if we could retain, or regain, our sense of humor and a spirit of playfulness as we age, life would be more tolerable and pleasurable, even though it might still be difficult.

So don't be afraid to have fun and to take time to seek out those things that give you real pleasure. Try to meet life with a positive attitude, and learn to laugh more. Attitude can make the difference between an unhappy life and a vibrant and exciting life.

Senator Strom Thurmond, the oldest member of Congress at age 95, summed up his philosophy for a long life when he said: "The secret to long life is good diet, exercise, and an optimistic attitude." At age 90, Senator Thurmond exercised 50 minutes a day (calisthenics, swimming, bicycling, or lifting weights), avoided alcohol, caffeine, and fried foods.

We could all learn a lot from the 80, 90, and 100 year olds that continue to live happy and productive lives.

NEED MORE INFORMATION?

- The American Association of Retired Persons: 601 E. Street NW Washington, DC 20049: (202) 434-3525
- The American Association of Homes and Services for the Aging (provides free brochures on housing, how to choose a nursing home, independent living, continuing-care retirement communities, etc.): (202) 783-2242
- The Alzheimer's Association: 1-800-272-3900.
- Arthritis Foundation Information Hotline: 1-800-283-7800
- The Eldercare locator (helps with referrals to local caregiving organizations): 1-800-677-1116.
- The National Association for Area Agencies on Aging (offers nationwide directory assistance service to help connect caregivers with local support resources): 1-800-677-1116.
- The National Academy of Elder Law Attorneys (offers free brochures on medical decision making, long-term care insurance, living trusts, guardianship, how to find an elder-law attorney, etc.): (520) 881-4005.
- National Institute on Aging Information Center: 1-800-222-2225
- National Rehabilitation Information center (guides for researchers,

- families, and individuals with disabilities): 1-800-346-2742, or http://www.naric.com/naric
- U.S. Department of Health + Human Services (free copy of "Depression is a Treatable Illness"): 1-800-222-2225 (Supplies limited).
- Simon Foundation for Continence: 1-800-237-4666.
- American Association of Retired Persons (AARP): http://www.aarp.org/
- ElderHostel (college education for older adults): http://www.elderhostel.org/
- National Senior Services Corps (SS and older national volunteer programs): http://www.crs.gov/senior-a-html
- The Resource Directory for Older People (government agencies and resource centers on aging): http://www.aoa.dhhs.gov/aoa/resource.html

A REAL LIFE EXAMPLE OF SOMEONE WHO CHOSE

Kate Mathews, at age 30, re-evaluated her overall lifestyle. Even though she was not overweight and she was involved in regular dance classes, Kate felt her smoking and social drinking habits compromised her overall health. So, she stopped smoking and decided to make some other changes in her life. She restricted her drinking and reduced her consumption of meat, eggs, and high fat foods. She diversified her exercise program to include yoga, stretching, weights, walking, and bicycling (eventually biking 475 miles on the Natchez Trace Parkway, at age 41, with her husband, Bob). Today, Kate and her husband live in the country, where they continue their healthy lifestyle, while working toward raising much of their own food, and enjoying the therapeutic effects of living closer to nature.

"I really believe that exercise and healthy eating today, at age 45, are an investment in my future good health, at age 85."

- Kate Mathews
Editor, Lark Books

WHAT DO I NEED TO DO?

*** Start exercising and eating nutritious foods as early in life as possible.
*** Include weight training in your exercise program, along with aerobic activity and stretching.
*** Maintain a positive attitude, and a sense of humor.
*** Don't classify yourself and your activities according to your age, but remember you are "as old as you feel."
*** Look at old age as an opportunity to have more time to improve your health and to do the things you have always wanted to do.
*** Simplify your life.

A THOUGHT TO REMEMBER

Many individuals have found their niche in life at the age of 70, 80, 90, and even 100 years of age. Your youth and your middle years have provided you with a wide range of wisdom, skills, and knowledge. Add boldness in your later years to your many talents and pursue your dreams!

CHAPTER 13

KEEPING WELLNESS SIMPLE

If you really want to know how to keep wellness simple, here it is:

1. YOU are responsible for your own health.

2. Since more than 50 percent of disease, disability, and death is caused by things we can control, you can cut your risks of illness and premature death by changing poor health habits.

3. These are good health habits you should incorporate into your life:

   - don't use tobacco
   - decrease the fat in your diet and eat at least 5 fruits and vegetables each day
   - exercise daily
   - don't misuse alcohol
   - keep preventive shots and vaccines up-to-date
   - avoid exposure to toxic substances
   - keep guns secure, or get rid of them
   - be sexually faithful to one uninfected partner
   - obey traffic laws & use protective devices such as seat belts, airbags, child restraint seats, & cycle helmets
   - don't use illegal drugs

- learn to deal with stress
- cultivate strong relationships
- avoid poverty
- live where you have access to health services
- accident-proof your life
- develop a sense of humor
- get sufficient sleep
- eat less
- have a pet
- enjoy nature
- keep your surroundings quiet & peaceful
- balance your life
- cultivate moral & spiritual wellness
- seek knowledge & educate yourself
- wash your hands

4. Stay positive as you age. Old age does not mean you have to be weak and sick. Emphasis on regular weight-bearing exercise, such as walking, plus weight training and stretching, along with the preceding good health habits will help keep you mobile and flexible even into your 80's and 90's.

> **In other words, exercise, eat right, live a peaceful and respectful existence with other people and the world around you, rest when you are tired, keep your life as simple as possible, seek spiritual strength, act with honesty and kindness, avoid unnatural substances, be careful enough to avoid accidents, and love life as much as possible. This will not only decrease your health risks, but it will magnify the quality of your life, and leave the world a better place for your existence.**

PERSONAL NOTE FROM THE AUTHOR

In our country, where 42 million adults and 10 million children are not insured, where 34 million Americans suffer from chronic pain, where 5 million children take medicine or inhale sprays, and where one trillion dollars was spent on healthcare in 1997, it is obvious we must take more individual responsibility for our health. That is why I wrote this book, and I sincerely hope this book has been of help to you. My prayers and best wishes go with you as you attempt to make changes in your life that will allow you to live longer, healthier, and happier. Life can be so much more livable and fun when we feel good and have a minimum amount of conflict to deal with.

The key to any endeavor is perseverance. So, don't get discouraged if you fail here and there. If you continue to try, and if you learn from your mistakes, you will eventually get to your goal.

The search for good health is a timeless one, recognized by men and women through the ages as a necessary ingredient for happiness. This truth was stated beautifully by John Locke in 1693 when he said, "A sound mind in a sound body, is a short but full description of a happy state in this world."

In one sentence, John Locke has pretty much covered what it has taken a whole book for me to say. So, let me close with one last thought for you: as you change your life, be sure and celebrate your accomplishments and victories...and good luck, and God bless your journey.